Current Advances and Future Trends in Vascular Neurology

Editor

MICHAEL J. SCHNECK

NEUROLOGIC CLINICS

www.neurologic.theclinics.com

Consulting Editor
RANDOLPH W. EVANS

August 2024 • Volume 42 • Number 3

ELSEVIER

1600 John F. Kennedy Boulevard ● Suite 1800 ● Philadelphia, Pennsylvania, 19103-2899

http://www.theclinics.com

NEUROLOGIC CLINICS Volume 42, Number 3
August 2024 ISSN 0733-8619, ISBN-13: 978-0-323-93865-5

Editor: Stacy Eastman
Developmental Editor: Varun Gopal

Neurologic Clinics (ISSN 0733-8619) is published quarterly by Elsevier Inc., 360 Park Avenue South, New York, NY 10010–1710. Months of issue are February, May, August, and November. Periodicals postage paid at New York, NY, and additional mailing offices. Subscription prices are $360.00 per year for US individuals, $100.00 per year for US students, $445.00 per year for Canadian individuals, $504.00 per year for international individuals, $210.00 for foreign students/residents, and $100.00 for Canadian students/residents. For institutional access pricing please contact Customer Service via the contact information below. To receive student/resident rate, orders must be accompanied by name of affiliated institution, date of term, and the *signature* of program/residency coordinator on institution letterhead. Orders will be billed at individual rate until proof of status is received. Foreign air speed delivery is included in all *Clinics* subscription prices. All prices are subject to change without notice. **POSTMASTER:** Send address changes to *Neurologic Clinics*, Elsevier Health Sciences Division, Subscription Customer Service, 3251 Riverport Lane, Maryland Heights, MO 63043. **Customer Service: Telephone: 1-800-654-2452 (U.S. and Canada); 314-447-8871 (outside U.S. and Canada). Fax: 314-447-8029. E-mail: journalscustomerservice-usa@elsevier.com (for print support); journalsonlinesupport-usa@elsevier.com (for online support).**

Reprints. For copies of 100 or more of articles in this publication, please contact the Commercial Reprints Department, Elsevier Inc., 360 Park Avenue South, New York, New York, 10010-1710; Tel.: +1-212-633-3874; Fax: +1-212-633-3820, and E-mail: reprints@elsevier.com.

Neurologic Clinics is also published in Spanish by Nueva Editorial Interamericana S.A., Mexico City, Mexico.

Neurologic Clinics is covered in *Current Contents/Clinical Medicine, MEDLINE/PubMed (Index Medicus), EMBASE/Excerpta Medica,* and *PsycINFO,* and *ISI/BIOMED.*

Contributors

CONSULTING EDITOR

RANDOLPH W. EVANS, MD
Clinical Professor, Department of Neurology, Baylor College of Medicine, Houston, Texas, USA

EDITOR

MICHAEL J. SCHNECK, MD
Professor, Neurology and Neurosurgery, Loyola University Chicago Stritch School of Medicine, Maywood, Illinois, USA

AUTHORS

SAEED ABDOLLAHIFARD, MD
Senior Researcher, School of Medicine, Shiraz University of Medical Sciences, Research Center for Neuromodulation and Pain, Shiraz, Iran

RICHARD A. BERNSTEIN, MD, PhD
Professor, Northwestern University Feinberg School of Medicine, Chicago, Illinois, USA

FAN Z. CAPRIO, MD
Associate Professor, Northwestern University Feinberg School of Medicine, Chicago, Illinois, USA

AMIRMOHAMMAD FARROKHI, MD
Junior Researcher, School of Medicine, Shiraz University of Medical Sciences, Shiraz, Iran

BRANDI R. FRENCH, MD
Professor of Neurology, University of Missouri Columbia School of Medicine, Columbia, Missouri, USA

RAJEEV K. GARG, MD, MS
Associate Professor, Division of Critical Care Neurology, Section of Cognitive Neurosciences, Rush University Medical Center, Chicago, Illinois, USA

CAMILO R. GOMEZ, MD, MBA
Professor of Neurology, University of Missouri Columbia School of Medicine, Columbia, Missouri, USA

FRANCISCO E. GOMEZ, MD
Assistant Professor of Neurology, University of Missouri Columbia School of Medicine, Columbia, Missouri, USA

NITIN GOYAL, MD
Neurointensivist, Neurointerventionalist, Semmes Murphey Clinic; Assistant Professor, Departments of Neurology and Neurosurgery, University of Tennessee Health Science Center, Memphis, Tennessee, USA

VIOLIZA INOA, MD
Vascular Neurologist, Neurointerventionalist, Semmes Murphey Clinic; Associate Professor, Departments of Neurology and Neurosurgery, University of Tennessee Health Science Center, Memphis, Tennessee, USA

GIUSEPPE LANZINO, MD
Neurosurgeon, Departments of Neurological Surgery and Radiology, Mayo Clinic, Rochester, Minnesota, USA

ENRIQUE C. LEIRA, MD, MS
Professor, Departments of Neurology, Neurosurgery, and Epidemiology, University of Iowa Carver College of Medicine, Iowa City, Iowa, USA

DAVID S. LIEBESKIND, MD
Director, UCLA Department of Neurology, Neurovascular Imaging Research Core, UCLA Comprehensive Stroke Center, University of California Los Angeles (UCLA), Los Angeles, California, USA

ASHKAN MOWLA, MD, FAHA, FAAN
Assistant Professor, Division of Stroke and Endovascular Neurosurgery, Department of Neurological Surgery, Keck School of Medicine, University of Southern California (USC), Los Angeles, California, USA

RYAN T. MUIR, MD
Resident Physician, Calgary Stroke Program, Departments of Clinical Neurosciences and Community Health Sciences, University of Calgary, Hotchkiss Brain Institute, Calgary, Alberta, Canada

ADNAN I. QURESHI, MD
Professor of Neurology, University of Missouri Columbia School of Medicine, Columbia, Missouri, USA

ALEJANDRO A. RABINSTEIN, MD
Neurologist, Department of Neurology, Mayo Clinic, Rochester, Minnesota, USA

HANNAH J. ROEDER, MD, MPH
Clinical Assistant Professor, Department of Neurology, University of Iowa Carver College of Medicine, Iowa City, Iowa, USA

ERIC E. SMITH, MD, MPH
Professor, Calgary Stroke Program, Departments of Clinical Neurosciences and Community Health Sciences, University of Calgary, Hotchkiss Brain Institute, Calgary, Alberta, Canada

CHRISTINE E. YEAGER, MD
Assistant Professor, Division of Critical Care Neurology, Rush University Medical Center, Chicago, Illinois, USA

MARGARET Y. YU, MD
Clinical Assistant Professor, University of Illinois at Chicago, Chicago, Illinois, USA

Contents

> Artificial intelligence (AI) is currently being used as a routine tool for day-to-day activity. Medicine is not an exception to the growing usage of AI in various scientific fields. Vascular and interventional neurology deal with diseases that require early diagnosis and appropriate intervention, which are crucial to saving patients' lives. In these settings, AI can be an extra pair of hands for physicians or in conditions where there is a shortage of clinical experts. In this article, the authors have reviewed the common metrics used in interpreting the performance of models and common algorithms used in this field.

> Cardioembolism accounts globally for around 25% of ischemic strokes and is more often associated with higher rates of morbidity and mortality. Potential sources of cardioembolism into the intracranial circulation include paradoxic embolism, dysrhythmias, structural heart disease, and valvular heart disease. To identify the etiology of a patient's ischemic stroke, thorough investigation of the intracardiac structures, assessment of dysrhythmias, and consideration of high-risk events such as cardiac surgery are crucial. Treatment after cardioembolic stroke can be personalized based on the underlying cardioembolic source to minimize the risk of recurrent cerebral ischemic events.

> Cerebral small vessel disease (CSVD) is a spectrum of disorders that affect small arterioles, venules, cortical and leptomeningeal vessels, perivascular spaces, and the integrity of neurovascular unit, blood brain barrier, and surrounding glia and neurons. CSVD is an important cause of lacunar ischemic stroke and sporadic hemorrhagic stroke, as well as dementia–which will constitute some of the most substantive population and public health challenges over the next century. This article provides an overview of updated pathophysiologic frameworks of CSVD; discusses common and underappreciated clinical and neuroimaging manifestations of CSVD; and reviews emerging genetic risk factors linked to sporadic CSVD.

Spontaneous intracerebral hemorrhage accounts for approximately 10% to 15% of all strokes in the United States and remains one of the deadliest. Of concern is the increasing prevalence, especially in younger populations. This article reviews the following: epidemiology, risk factors, outcomes, imaging findings, medical management, and updates to surgical management.

Major advances in neurocritical care and the modalities used to treat aneurysms have led to improvement in the outlook of patients with aneurysmal subarachnoid hemorrhage. Yet, several knowledge gaps remain widely open. Variability in practices stems from the lack of solid evidence to guide management, which recent guidelines from professional organizations aim to mitigate. In this article, the authors review some of these gaps in knowledge, highlight important messages from recent management guidelines, emphasize aspects of our practice that we consider particularly useful to optimize patient outcomes, and suggest future areas of research.

Neuroendovascular rescue of patients with acute ischemic stroke caused by a large arterial occlusion has evolved throughout the first quarter of the present century, and continues to do so. Starting with the intra-arterial instillation of thrombolytic agents via microcatheters to dissolve occluding thromboembolic material, the current status is one that includes a variety of different techniques such as direct aspiration of thrombus, removal by stent retriever, adjuvant techniques such as balloon angioplasty, stenting, and tactical intra-arterial instillation of thrombolytic agents in smaller branches to treat no-reflow phenomenon. The results have been consistently shown to benefit these patients, irrespective of whether they had already received intravenous tissue-type plasminogen activator or not. Improved imaging methods of patient selection and tactically optimized periprocedural care measures complement this dimension of the practice of neurointervention.

The article summarizes the training pathways and vocational opportunities within the field of vascular neurology. It highlights the groundbreaking clinical trials that transformed acute stroke care and the resultant increased demand for readily available vascular neurology expertise. The article emphasizes the need to train a larger number of diverse physicians in the subspecialty and the role of vascular neurologists in improving outcomes across demographic and geographic lines.

Role of Stroke Scales and Scores in Cerebrovascular Disease

Violiza Inoa and Nitin Goyal

This article provides a comprehensive review of widely utilized stroke scales in both routine clinical settings and research. These scales are crucial for planning treatment, predicting outcomes, and helping stroke patients recover. They also play a pivotal role in planning, executing, and comprehending stroke clinical trials. Each scale presents distinct advantages and limitations, and the authors explore these aspects within the article. The authors' intention is to provide the reader with practical insights for a clear understanding of these scales, and their effective use in their clinical practice.

NEUROLOGIC CLINICS

ISSUES OF RELATED INTEREST

Neurosurgery Clinics
https://www.neurosurgery.theclinics.com/
Neuroimaging Clinics
https://www.neuroimaging.theclinics.com/
Psychiatric Clinics
https://www.psych.theclinics.com/
Child and Adolescent Psychiatric Clinics
https://www.childpsych.theclinics.com/

THE CLINICS ARE AVAILABLE ONLINE!
Access your subscription at:
www.theclinics.com

Performance Metrics, Algorithms, and Applications of Artificial Intelligence in Vascular and Interventional Neurology

A Review of Basic Elements

Saeed Abdollahifard, MD[a,b], Amirmohammad Farrokhi, MD[a], Ashkan Mowla, MD[c], David S. Liebeskind, MD[d,*]

KEYWORDS

- Neurology • Interventional neurology • Artificial intelligence • AI
- Performance metrics • Vascular neurology

KEY POINTS

- An overview of artificial intelligence (AI) and its specific use in vascular and interventional neurology, and its implications is explored and explained in this article.
- The key presenting factors of AI models, their metrics, is thoroughly discussed with a notion to how these factors may be misleading as well as how they help us evaluate their performance.
- There have been numerous models deployed and developed since the initial introduction of AI, of which a sufficient number and how they operate is illustrated.
- The specific application of AI models in each aspect and sub-category of vascular and interventional neurology is presented with regards to how these models prove useful independently or with junction to clinicians as their assistant.
- *AI should be regarded as any other tool created in the human history and its use should be carefully practiced with regards to its implications, advantages, shortcomings, and determined target.*

[a] School of Medicine, Shiraz University of Medical Sciences, Shiraz, Iran; [b] Research Center for Neuromodulation and Pain, Shiraz, Iran; [c] Division of Stroke and Endovascular Neurosurgery, Department of Neurological Surgery, Keck School of Medicine, University of Southern California (USC), Los Angeles, CA, USA; [d] UCLA Department of Neurology, Neurovascular Imaging Research Core, UCLA Comprehensive Stroke Center, University of California Los Angeles(UCLA), CA, USA
* Corresponding author. 635 Charles E Young Drive, South, Los Angeles, CA 90049.
E-mail address: davidliebeskind@yahoo.com

Neurol Clin 42 (2024) 633–650
https://doi.org/10.1016/j.ncl.2024.03.001
0733-8619/24/© 2024 Elsevier Inc. All rights reserved.

neurologic.theclinics.com

INTRODUCTION

Artificial intelligence (AI) has become the topic of interest in various fields of research in the current century, especially in recent years, engulfing many aspects of our lives ranging from daily activities such as shopping and social interactions to complex decision-making systems in medical sciences and predicting the needs of major industries.[1–3] Medical sciences and medicine have been of the slowest fields to adopt and accept the use of AI in their practice since the introduction of AI in the 1950s, primarily due to problems in the limitations setting a different path between computer and logic problems and medical problems.[4] With the further development of AI, the emergence of deep learning (DL) models, and the existence of more potent efficient graphics processing units allowing a much higher processing power, the fundamental issues surrounding the applicability and availability of models that are both reliable and efficient in medical fields were overcome in the twentieth century, and since then, there is an explosive, day-to-day advancement in the application of AI in medicine.[2,4,5] Neurology and neurologic surgery serve as no exception to this flood of novel technology, and countless studies have proven the applicability and usefulness of AI in numerous aspects of these fields. As these fields include practices from imaging and screening studies to decision-making regarding the choice of proper treatment protocol all the way through outcome evaluation and post-treatment care optimization, proper and informed development and use of AI models are without a doubt beneficial to practitioners, patients, and the micromanagement and macromanagement of health care ecosystems.[6] Current studies have utilized models for a variety of uses, such as image-processing models to diagnose, detect, and segment intracranial and intraspinal lesions and the outcome of traumatic brain injury patients, natural language processing to evaluate large texts in medical records, and many other fields.[7–13] Despite the apparent promise of integration of AI models in all aspects of life, the so-called "hope," there is concern regarding the interpretability and explainability of such models, causing a generalized "hype" toward the applicability of AI models in all aspects of a field. These issues can be properly addressed via the development of policies already at hand, like explainable AI.[14] In addition to this general concern toward AI models, proper orientation of developers and users of such models can propose a more informed application and development strategies.[15] This solution includes proper choice of problems (ie, scenarios in which AI models come to aid us), proper choice of models as solutions, use of a unified, fluent terminology, and a realistic understanding of outcome measures of each model such as precision, recall, and the area under the receiver operating characteristic (ROC) curve (AUC).[16,17]

METRICS

Evaluation metrics of a model are the basic concept for assessing the performance of the model. Hence, it is important to first discuss the definition of these terms and what they actually mean in regard to clinical practice.

Confusion Matrix

A confusion matrix is an N × N matrix in which N represents the number of predicted classes. It can be 2 when our targeted outcome is true or false while processing image data or when assessing the true or falseness of a result, called a binary outcome. The number of classes can be more when discussing multiple class outcomes such as low, medium, and high risk. Confusion matrices are amongst the most basic and commonly used concepts, and researchers may be familiar with the topic since the same rule applies to statistical analysis. A number of outcome measures can be calculated using the confusion matrix as follows:[18]

True positive: It is the rate of outcomes calculated as positive, and it matches the real data measures.

True negative: It is the rate of outcomes calculated as negative, and it matches the real data measures.

False positive: It is the rate of outcomes falsely calculated as positive.

False negative: It is the rate of outcomes falsely calculated as negative.

		Actual Results	
		Positive	Negative
Predicted Results	Positive	True positive	False positive
	Negative	False negative	True negative

These 4 actually do not serve as metrics but as basic data interpreted from the confusion matrix. In a matrix with N > 2, the total incorrect outcome values in positive and negative tables sum up to make the respective false positive and negative counts.

Accuracy: It is the rate of total correct calculated outcomes divided by the total calculated outcomes.

Sensitivity (recall): It is the rate of correctly identified positive outcomes to all correct positive values.

Specificity: It is the rate of correctly identified negative outcomes to all correct negative values.

Positive predictive value (PPV) (precision): It is the rate of correctly identified positive outcomes to all positive outcome predictions.

Negative predictive value (NPV): It is the rate of correctly identified negative outcomes to all negative outcome predictions.

Metric	Calculation
Accuracy	$\dfrac{TP+TN}{TP+TN+FP+FN}$
Sensitivity (recall)	$\dfrac{TP}{TP+FN}$
Specificity	$\dfrac{TN}{TN+FP}$
Positive predictive value (PPV) (precision)	$\dfrac{TP}{TP+FP}$
Negative predictive value (NPV)	$\dfrac{TN}{TN+FN}$

These metrics are conventionally used and illustrate a clear, though basic, overview of the performance of any model regardless of its purpose or architecture.[19] Accuracy, though it may look informative and simple, has several shortcomings. First, it is susceptible to the number of cases allocated in each category. An unbalanced dataset having too many positives or negatives can lean into overclassifying data into the over-weighted category, and even though having a high accuracy rate, the model falls short of identifying the less-weighted category and still shows a high accuracy rate. This problem can escalate and become completely misleading in multi-class problems, with 1 specific class having comparatively more and one having majorly less count.

This leads us to reside to more specific outcome measures and further understand them as we move along. The next outcome measure widely used both in statistics and AI is sensitivity. Sensitivity shows the number of positive outcomes predicted divided by total positive values. More commonly labeled as recall in literature, sensitivity serves as a sufficient measure to evaluate how well the model performs in identifying the correct cases. However, negative outcomes are not illustrated in this measure, and a model can overclassify positive cases in order to maintain a high recall rate. Specificity demonstrates the rate of correctly identified negative outcomes to true negative values. The same rule applies since the overclassification of negative outcomes falsely increases the specificity rate without any improvement in the model's applicability. Sensitivity and specificity combined, however, have served as a reliable index of the performance of models and priorly in fields such as diagnostic tests. One may prefer sensitivity in screening tests since the detection of cases with a certain pathology is favored on a large scale with regard to the cost and importance of identifying the target. In another setup, specificity is preferred when wrongly identifying a case as positive could lead to impactful effects such as emotional and psychological burden and high costs for follow-up and further workup. These concepts have evolved into the AI paradigm, signifying the importance of correctly identifying positive or negative outcomes depending on the problem and the solution. Even though the combination of these 2 metrics can be useful, the lack of a singular outcome measure to overview the performance of the model still exists. Another evaluation metric is the positive predictive value. As the name suggests, this metric shows the value of a positive prediction by the model or, more specifically, the rate of true positives divided by all positively predicted values by the model. Also called precision, this metric leans to denote how well the model has identified its positive cases. Similar to recall, precision is biased toward the positive outcome even though it includes false positives instead of false negatives. NPV signifies the rate of which negative outcomes predicted are true, that is, the rate of true negatives divided by true and false negatives. PPVs and NPVs can be used in combination in a similar fashion as that of sensitivity and specificity, with their main difference being the emphasis on the model outcome evaluation on the former since the denominator is the model's prediction result in contrast to the latter, which uses the true results as the denominator. The same concern applies to PPVs and NPVs since these 2 metrics do not combine to create a singular metric. These basic concepts may appear basic, but their usage to represent any model's performance may prove to be either an accessory to further understand the plus sides of a model and to understand its weaknesses in parallel or misleading since models that are biased toward a certain category or class can have some rather excellent metrics regarding the biased side without achieving reasonable applicability and reliability.[20] With the mentioned concern regarding the lack of a singular metric, the F1 score becomes rather necessary to understand and mention since it is a harmonic mean of precision and recall with the formula as follows:

$$F1\ Score = \frac{2}{Precision^{-1} + Recall^{-1}} = 2 \times \frac{Precision \times Recall}{Precision + Recall} = \frac{2 \times TP}{2 \times TP + FP + FN}$$

The use of harmonic mean instead of an arithmetical mean (commonly named "mean" plainly) furtherly emphasizes the extremes of a value range, usually misunderstood while using the arithmetical mean. A simple example would be if a model has a precision rate of 0% and a recall rate of 100%, the arithmetical mean would be 50%, and if precision alone is represented as a metric, the performance may look significant with a mean of 50%. In the real setup though, it can belong to a classifier wrongly predicting only 1 category as output. In this setup, the F1 score is 0, more accurately illustrating the model's inability to correctly identify any category except the target in a binary classification problem. It can be deduced that the F1 score overcomes 1 issue by including both false negative and false positive predictions of the model (precision includes false positives, and recall includes false negatives).[21] Since there have been challenges primarily accepting the AI models as reliable tools to aid clinicians and to apply them in clinical settings, the primary goal of introducing AI models to these settings has been proving them useful and "correct" regarding problems raised. F1 score serves best as a solution to this problem, illustrating a harmonic mean of how the model performed regarding true positives in the context of false positives and negatives. It should be highly noted that even if this metric outperforms the priors, it still emphasizes the true positive counts and could be biased, even though logically less than others, toward a model identifying positive outcomes in a biased manner.[22] A more advanced metric suggested to be applied in binary classification problems is the Matthews correlation coefficient (MCC) or phi coefficient, which is defined identically to Pearson's phi coefficient and is calculated as follows:

$$MCC = \frac{TP \times TN - FP \times FN}{\sqrt{(TP+FP)(TP+FN)(TN+FP)(TN+FN)}}$$

Its value ranges from -1 to $+1$ ranging from extremely poor to extremely well prediction, respectively. It is significantly noteworthy since it includes all parts of a confusion matrix in its calculation, lowering the effect of data imbalance in the calculation of the metric.[23] It has also generalized into multi-class problems as the R_k statistical.

The Receiver Operating Characteristic Curve

Moving a little distant from straight calculations from the confusion matrix, it should be noted that most models represent their outcomes as probabilities of each case belonging to a classified outcome category. The cutoff point which the model decides whether a particular probability can suffice for a selected prediction to belong to a certain category is called the threshold. A model can achieve different metrics based on the variation of such threshold since it changes the predicted values when classified into categories. This illustrates the basic concept for ROC curve, which is a graphical plot showing the ability of a binary classifier while thresholds are varied, while the true positive rate (TPR) (sensitivity) is plotted against the false positive rate(1-specificity). The area under this curve, called the AUC, is calculated as a metric to decide whether a model can outperform a random decider, having a 50% AUC. AUC values of a model closer to 1 or 100% of the plot shows the model's more accurate prediction across thresholds and hence proves it more reliable. As the AUC approaches lower rates and closer to 50%, it can be deduced that the model's performance shows no difference to a random guesser, and hence it is impractical.[24] Unfortunately, there is no direct use of AUC in multi-class classification problems. The alternative is the evaluation of AUC in 2 manners, one versus one or one versus the rest.[18] Though it can provide helpful insight toward the performance of the model, variations in multiple classes and the models performance whilst regarding each category as the main target can be deceiving and precise attention to each and every AUC and ROC plotted in this setup is a necessity. Another alternative, AUC_μ, is a derivative of the original AUC formula based on the Mann-Whitney U statistical. This metric can be used as a novel approach to evaluate a model's outcome on multiclass classification in the same manner as AUC in binary classification problems.[25]

Log Loss

Furtherly digging into differences in models' architecture, algorithms such as logistic regression, gradient boosting, and random forest eventually provide us with probability outputs in contrast to support vector machines (SVMs) or k nearest neighbor, which provide a class output. This introduces a challenge of defining the best threshold for models with probability output and, in return, enables us to use dynamic metrics like AUC as mentioned earlier. Another metric to be considered is the log loss. It is defined by the negative average of the logarithm of predicted probabilities for each instance.

$$Log\ loss = -\frac{1}{N}\sum_{i=1}^{N} y_i \cdot \log(p(y_i)) + (1 - y_i) \cdot \log(1 - p(y_i))$$

where, $p(y_i)$ is the predicted probability of a positive class

$1-p(y_i)$ is the predicted probability of a negative class

$y_i = 1$ for the positive class and 0 for the negative class (actual values)

When plotted, the log loss declines as predictions improve. Naturally being a logarithmic function, the log loss increases drastically when probability approaches 0. It can be deduced that the lower the log loss of a model, the better its performance is in predicting the outcome. Interpreting log loss can prove to be difficult specifically in multi-class problems since the raw information provided by the plot and the sole number calculated may not be representative of the model's actual performance or its specific performance regarding 1 class outcome. However, using log loss in parallel to other metrics and with regard to the problem introduced and the model as the solution can furtherly illuminate the performance of the model. Another point could be made that log loss can be used to compare models proposed for a single problem.

Root Mean Squared Error and Root Mean Squared Logarithmic Error

One of the most popular metrics in regression problems, the root mean squared error (RMSE), is calculated as suggested by its name. It's a square root of the average of the squared differences between predictions and actual values. It includes an assumption of unbiased errors and normal distribution of errors. Since the formula encompasses squared roots, a large number of deviations are empowered. The squared error cancels the negative and positive errors, and it gives higher weights to errors compared to the mean absolute error (MAE). It should be noted that outlier data heavily affect the RMSE and it is advised to consider and remove such data to avoid overestimation of this metric. The root mean squared logarithmic error (RMSLE) takes the logarithm of prediction and actual values in order to escape the error of overcalculation when both the predicted and actual values are big numbers and, therefore their squared differences, even though small in comparison to the nature of data.

$$RMSE = \sqrt{\frac{1}{N}\sum_{i=1}^{N}(Predicted_i - Actual_i)^2}$$

$$RMSLE = \sqrt{\frac{1}{N}\sum_{i=1}^{N}(\log(Predicted_i+1) - \log(Actual_i+1))^2}$$

INTRODUCTION TO MACHINE LEARNING MODELS AND ALGORITHMS

Now that we have re-familiarized ourselves with the terminology used while reporting a model's performance, it is time to explore how this "black box" does the wonder of replicating human intelligence.[26] Though thoughts of a machine being able to imitate human intelligence grow all the way back to the tenth century BC and many theorizations existed ever since the first domino to fall perhaps could be Alan Turing's 1950 article "The Imitation Game" in which he raised the question "Can machines think?" and then he proposed the Turing test as a measure for machine intelligence.[27,28] The Dartmouth Summer Research Project on AI, held in 1956, is considered the event officially coining the term AI and founding the concept as it is followed into modern times.[29] Since then, AI has experienced several up and downs regarding prospect, applicability, funding, and computation power backing its development.[1,30] It can be stated that with the integration of computer systems into all aspects of life and the exponential growth in computational power, the twenty-first century marked the booming era for AI systems. DL, defined by the use of multiple layers in the model's network, started outperforming other models in the late 2000s, and with the introduction of novel algorithms using DL, a global transformation in AI occurred.[31–34] In parallel to evolutions in algorithms and model architecture, computer hardware has also improved drastically since 2010s and has enabled us to construct bigger and more complex functional models.[35] Nowadays, a versatile array of techniques and paradigms are available to conduct models under the umbrella term of AI.

Proper categorization of AI models can be challenging since many definitions may overlap or appear confusing. However, we try to categorize models based on how they operate and their applicability. One of the rather primary categorizations of models could be regarding how they become trained, the process in which a naïve model becomes able to perform certain tasks as designated. The 3 main types of this process, also called learning, consist of 3 main types: supervised, unsupervised, and semi-supervised learning.[36]

Note: Not all AI models use learning (eg, good old-fashioned AI or basic natural language processing models). However, since most proficient models nowadays are amongst machine learning (ML) models, it is safe to say most models we encounter use a grade of learning.

The so-called "supervision" used in this nomenclature is attributed to the contribution of a human counterpart to train or teach the model. In more comprehendible terms, a model is supervised when the input data and outputs used for training the model are already labeled by a human, so the algorithm would only compute the relations between the input data and the outcome provided.[37,38] Unsupervised models, on the contrary, consist of models training themselves to find certain relations, patterns, or distinctions between the input data.[39] Semi-supervised models use a fusion of both these learning algorithms where the training of the algorithm is assisted by labeling the data by a human interpreter in some points and left to the algorithms themselves in other points.[40] Logically speaking, since unsupervised models do not have an endpoint appointed to them via the operator, they serve best in categorization or pattern identification in larger datasets where individual data labeling has a large cost or burden.[41–43] However, supervised models may provide better outcomes in tasks such as predictions or detections of a specific endpoint.[44] The choice of each learning process is a delicate task-dependent in each project, availability of resources and data, and consideration of cost both tolled on human researchers and the models regarding computational power and time required for the learning process.[45] It is worth mentioning that there is a general tendency toward the use of supervised learning models since they have proven to provide more efficient outcomes regarding specific problems introduced in the field of medicine.[46,47] Unsupervised models can be used instead as sources of preliminary classification and categorization algorithms developed on larger scale data, identifying patterns in a bigger scheme.[48,49]

Supervised models, in turn, consist of numerous algorithms and approaches. One of the main divisions of supervised models can be considered as regression and classification models.[50] Regression models are usually used when there is a direct relationship between the input data and the outcome. It can be used to predict continuous variables such as laboratory reports, length of hospital stay, and duration of admission.[50,51] Variates of regressors such as linear regression, Bayesian linear regression, and regression trees are models applied for this problem. Classification problems occur when the outcome is categorical.[52] Even though we encounter many scenarios in real life where the outcome, though categorical, consists of multiple outcomes, most models implemented are to solve binary categorical problems. It is proven that an increase in outcome categories which leads to a multi-class classification problem instead of a binary classification problem decreases the model's performance and efficiency.[53] Hence, it is preferred to reduce problems to binary classification problems. Decision trees, SVMs, and random forests are among the other models used for solving classification problems.

Unsupervised models also consist of different approaches. They can be categorized into models devoted to clustering or association rules. Clustering focuses on grouping objects into clusters with the most similarities and distinguishing them from other groups based on their differences.[54,55] Association rules, on the other hand, try to find relationships between variables in a more linear way. As clustering models try to divide the data and label them based on similarities found by the model, associative models tend to find co-occurring instances to create relations in the input data.[56] K-means clustering, k-nearest neighbors, hierarchal clustering, and apriori algorithm are models implemented as solutions to clustering and associating problems.

Artificial neural networks (ANNs) are a broad branch of ML models based on neural networks existing in biological brains. ANNs are based on an interconnected network of artificial neurons, also called nodes, which tend to basically resemble biological neurons. The interactions between these neurons, called edges, vaguely imitate neuronal synapses with an adjustable weight to the input values based on its learning algorithm. This weight increases or decreases the value of the input, and when the input crosses a certain amount, called the threshold, the artificial neuron gets triggered. Neurons are eventually aggregated into layers, and data entered in the input model cross multiple layers from the first input layer to the last layer, called the output layer. The weights and thresholds mentioned are altered by the algorithm until they reach an optimum point.[57–59] Variations in the basic structure of ANNs have led to the evolution of newer algorithms such as convolutional neural networks (CNNs), recurrent neural networks (RNNs), and deep neural networks (DNNs).[60] DNN, also a general term regarding its concept, applies the use of multiple "deep" layers in the network architecture.[61] RNNs use a recurrent architecture type, as the name suggests, constructing a bidirectional array with nodes affecting other nodes in previous layers in addition to the conventional feedforward architecture.[61] The latter using the feedforward neural network architecture, a more basic form of ANNs in which only there is a flow of data toward the last layer and no backward data transfer occurs. CNNs apply convolution in at least 1 of their layers, using this mathematical manipulation instead of basic matrix multiplication, these models based on CNN architecture have had a major impact on image processing tasks and computer vision. Various implementations of CNNs have aided physicians in the detection and segmentation tasks in medical imaging.[62,63]

One of the most important notes to be taken from this mixture of architectures, paradigms, and methods to use in the field of AI is that regardless of its novelty, complexity, or intended design, a model should be specifically and thoughtfully chosen in order to achieve the optimum performance intended for a single problem.[64] It can be deduced that with further and deeper study of each of the architectures mentioned earlier, a number of solutions would be available once a problem proposes itself. The crucial factor of picking the best solution becomes a complex question itself since it does not encompass simply applying a mysterious "black box" as a solution.[65] Important factors surrounding the problem regarding data size, availability of human counterparts to label the dataset in order to achieve supervised learning, and computational power are amongst the most basic questions one should answer before being able to consider the best algorithm as the solution.[66] It is also key to approach this matter as a complete project where there are numerous routes and points where pitfalls and misunderstandings can occur.[67] Poor choice of a model, improper data handling and labeling leading to false or corrupted data, insufficient or oversized data size, improper pre-processing, and wrongful interpretation of the output and performance metrics pointed at before are among the main issues regarding the use of AI models, sometimes wrongfully picked as the easier solution to problems.[68–71]

Data pre-processing: This is the manipulation of data to enhance a model's performance. It ranges from simply dropping improper data to data cleansing, data editing, and overall examination of data regarding falsely recorded records.

Data post-processing: This is the further processing of the information extracted by a process to evaluate its output, metrics, and overall meaning of the result. This step can utilize cautionary, logical analysis of the outcome and results of a model.

Fuzzy Logic

Fuzzy logic is a form of reasoning system allowing a multi-graded fashion of true and false. It can be represented as a mathematical way to represent uncertainty in decision-making, a scenario well-known in the medical sciences.[72] Fuzzy logic differs from AI since it is basically a reasoning method based on human decision-making which is based on a non-numeric sense implicated by them. Fuzzy logic implementation basically consists of converting the crisp input data to fuzzy sets called fuzzification, creating a rule base implying how any quality of input leads to next outcome, an inference engine determining how the current input and output duo matches the set rules and combining them to construct a reasoning model, and finally the defuzzification to convert the fuzzy sets into crisp data.[73] Fuzzy logic has been implemented in various fields of medicine so far, and its uncanny resemblance to human logic, in addition to its ability to fuse into AI models, can paint it as a promising field of study.[73–76]

APPLICATION OF ARTIFICIAL INTELLIGENCE MODELS IN THE FIELD OF VASCULAR AND INTERVENTIONAL NEUROLOGY
Stroke

Although the mortality rate from stroke has decreased by approximately 2.3% from 2005 to 2015, it is still the fifth leading cause of death in the United States.[77,78] Early diagnosis and intervention are considered to be necessary because as time passes, less tissue can be rescued, and treatment might be less effective.[79,80] However, the detection of stroke might be challenging, especially using non-contrast computed tomography (CT) scan, where the white matter-grey matter differentiation might be subtle in the first hours after stroke.[81] Also, making the decision to treat patients should be individualized, and discrepancies exist between imaging studies and the clinical condition of patients.[82] ML has emerged as an invaluable tool for physicians, providing an extra pair of hands in assistance addressing these issues. ML algorithms have been applied to detect, classify, and segment ischemic stroke lesions.[83,84] Wong and coworkers[85] used U-Net to segment lesions of patients with acute ischemic stroke from diffusion-weighted imaging. Using data across 875 patients, the developed model reached the overall Dice score of 0.85 with a 95% confidence interval (CI) of 0.82 to 0.88. Another study by Giancardo and coworkers[86] compared the ischemic core estimation of a DL model and neurologists using CT angiography. The results showed that for an ischemic core threshold of 15 mL and more, the DL model had a higher AUC compared to physicians (the highest AUC for the DL model was 0.90, and for stroke expert neurologists, it was 0.82). Zeng and coworkers[87] conducted a meta-analysis on the prediction of the outcome of patients with large vessel occlusion for both conventional ML models (including random forest models, support vector machine, ANN, and decision tree) and DL models. The results revealed that conventional models could predict the modified Rankin Scale (mRS) as an indicator of the function of patients with a pooled AUC of 0.81 and 95% CI (0.77–0.85) while DL models could predict good functional outcomes of patients (mRS 2 and less) with an AUC of 0.75 (95% CI: 0.70–0.81). Also, this study determined the overall AUC rate for successful reperfusion using the thrombolysis in cerebral infarction score for the aforementioned models and resulted in the pooled rate of 0.72 and (95% CI 0.56–0.88) from 3 conventional models and 0.65 (95% CI:0.62–0.68) from 1 DL model study. Another systematic review and meta-analysis was carried out by Wang and coworkers[88] to assess the performance of ML models for the prediction of infarct core using Dice similarity coefficient (DSC) score. The results demonstrated an overall DSC of 0.50 and a 95% CI of 0.39 to 0.61. In addition, subgroup analyses revealed that the best DSC will be achieved using DL models that are trained using CT data (DSC and 95% CI: 0.63 and 0.48–0.78). Hemorrhagic stroke is another type of stroke that may occur after intracerebral or subarachnoid hemorrhage (SAH) and accounts for a high rate of mortality and morbidity.[89,90] Consequently, along with other brain lesions, intracranial hemorrhage has been a point of interest for the development of AI models to do tasks such as the detection and prediction of outcomes.[91,92] Cortés-Ferre and coworkers[93] trained and tested a DL model based on ResNet using 752,799 scans. This model tried to identify patients with intracranial hemorrhages and reached an overall accuracy, TPR, true negative rate, PPV, and NPV of 100%, validating on an external data set consisting of scans of 55 patients. A study has been designed by Yun and coworkers[91] to address the question of whether the accuracy of physicians (radiologists, non-radiologist physicians, and neuroradiologists) will be increased with the aid of AI. They developed an AI model applying both a supervised and an unsupervised model consisting of a joint CNN-RNN model and an anomaly detection model, respectively, to detect intracranial hemorrhages. The results showed that the accuracy of physicians improved significantly with the aid of AI (97.03 vs 94.71 and P-value $P < .0001$). Tanioka and coworkers[94] tried to predict the expansion of hematoma in patients with acute intracerebral hemorrhage using several models and comparing them. Applying the k-nearest neighbors algorithms resulted in the best performance and could predict the hematoma expansion with an AUC of 0.790, a sensitivity of 84.6%, a specificity of 73.3%, and an accuracy of 77.5%. Three-model set was designed by Del Barrio and coworkers[95] to predict the prognosis of patients after intracranial hemorrhage in a binary classification manner. The study tested 3 models: a model trained using images (I-model), a model trained using tabular data(D-model), and a hybrid model. The hybrid model achieved the highest AUC of 0.924(95% CI: 0.831–0.986). Also, the I and D models held an AUC of 0.763 (95% CI: 0.622–0.902) and 0.746 (95% CI: 0.598–0.876), respectively. Although ML models showed promising outcomes, their usage may not always be successful and applicable. Rusche and coworkers[96] designed a study to compare the efficacy of 2 AI models of CNN and radiomics with human readers to investigate if ML could determine the onset of intracerebral hemorrhage more accurately than radiologists. The MAE for the CNN model was 9.77 hours (CI: 8.52–11.03 hours), for radiomics, it was 9.96 (CI: 8.68–11.32 hours) hours, and for human reader, it ranged from 11.21 to 13.38 hours. A major problem in detecting lesions is a low number of whole samples and small lesions that may lead to the underfitting of AI models. To overcome these issues, Zhang and coworkers[97] came up with a solution and generated intracranial lesions on CT scans to be used in the training of the AI models. They used artificial mask generators and lesion synthesis networks and robust AUC for intracranial hemorrhage detection from 84% to 91% and sensitivity for microbleeding from 49% to 70%.

Subdural Hematoma

Accompanying symptoms such as headache, limb weakness, malaise and memory impairment, subdural hematoma (SDH), and specifically chronic SDH (cSDH), a condition that,in some cases, needs interventions prior to inflicting major disabilities for the patients.[98,99] The mortality and morbidity rates of SDH are reported to be 0% to 32% and 0% to 25%, respectively.[100] The diagnosis is made by CT scan or MRI, and medical and surgical interventions, including embolization, would be the available treatment options based on the condition of patients.[101–103] As a result, the application of ML for imaging classifications and outcome prediction would be useful for physicians and related researchers. Colasurdo and coworkers[104] utilized a CNN architecture to detect SDH from non-contrast CT scans of patients. The results of external validation showed remarkable accuracy of 95.1(95% CI: 91.7%–97.3%), a sensitivity of 91.4% (95% CI: 82.3%–96.8%), and a specificity of 96.4% (95% CI 92.7%–98.5%). Also, this study tried to determine the maximum thickness of hematoma and midline shift that achieved MAE of 2.75 mm (95% CI 2.14–3.37 mm) and 0.93 mm (95% CI 0.55–1.31 mm), respectively. A meta-analysis was carried out by Abdollahifard and coworkers[9] to pool the overall rate of SDH detection/segmentation by DL models. The results analyzing 22 studies demonstrated that DL could perform this task at a sensitivity level of 88.8 to 86.8 and a specificity level of 97.2 to 86.9. A study designed by Biswas and coworkers[105] and tried multiple ML algorithms to predict the results of referral of cSDH patients in a binary manner (accept or reject for surgery) and trained their model on data of 1500 patients. The result revealed that ANN had the best performance in predicting the results with an accuracy of 96.2 (95% CI:94.4–97.7), a sensitivity of 92.19(95% CI: 87.5%–96.2%), a specificity of 98.0 (95% CI:95.6–99.2), and an AUC of 0.95(95% CI: 0.92–0.97). Also, the model performed well on external validation with an AUC of 0.896 (95% CI: 0.878–0.912) and accuracy of 92.2% (95% CI: 90.952–93.520). Extracting the feature importance in the trained ANN model showed that the size of the hematoma, age, and midline shift were the top 3 determinant factors. Applying these models in routine practice may decrease the workload for the health system and can play a role as a powerful assistant, especially for junior physicians. This model was made online to be used publicly. Another predictive model was developed by Zanaty and coworkers[106] to predict the recurrence of cSDH using data from

596 patients. Their optimal model achieved an accuracy of 93%, a precision of 84%, and a recall rate of 80%. In addition to the prediction of recurrence, Zanaty and coworkers[106] tried to test the model for predicting hospital stay and risk of stroke but the model was not performed well due to limitations according to the data. These results pointed out that for training and fitting an AI model properly, data preparation should carry out for each outcome prior to training the models.

Subarachnoid Hemorrhage

Vasospasm, re-bleeding, cerebral edema, and increase in intracranial pressure are complications of SAH and need urgent intervention to avoid a catastrophe. So, early detection and management of SAHs are vital and as a result, there is a growing body of evidence for applying AI as a predictive or detective model.[107–109] Nishi and coworkers[109] designed a study to see how effectively the DL model and human readers could diagnose SAH. The results showed that the model could detect lesions with an accuracy of 95% which was comparable with human readers (range from 96%–99%) consisting of neurosurgery specialists and non-specialists. A study by Thanellas and cowokers[110] deployed a DL model for the identification and localization of SAHs. The results in the external validation process demonstrated a sensitivity of 99.3% and a specificity of 63.2% for the detection task and a sensitivity of 87.4% and a specificity of 95.3% for the localization task among 2110 slices. A CNN model was trained by Kim and coworkers[111] to predict the risk of intracranial aneurysms rapture using data from 368 patients and then tested prospectively on 272 patients. The CNN model could predict the risk of rapture with a sensitivity of 78.76 (95% CI: 72.30%–84.30%), specificity of 72.15% (95% CI: 60.93%–81.65%), and an AUC of 0.75 (95% CI: 0.699%–0.805%) which was significantly higher than human reader with an AUC of 0.53 (96% CI: 0.47–0.59) and P-value < .001. Savarraj and coworkers[108] worked on an algorithm to assess the efficacy of ML models to predict the outcomes of patients with SAH, such as delayed cerebral ischemia and the functional outcome, which was defined as a binary outcome of mRS of 3 and less or 4 and more at the time of discharge and at the 3-month follow-up. The trained models yielded an overall AUC of 0.75(95% CI: 0.64–0.84) for the prediction of delayed cerebral ischemia and an AUC of 0.85(95% CI: 0.75–0.92) and 0.89 (95% CI: 0.81–0.94) for functional outcome at the time of discharge and at the follow-up, respectively. Jong and coworkers[112] developed a feedforward ANN to predict mortality during hospitalization, unfavorable mRS of more than 2 at the 6-month follow-up after discharge, and delayed cerebral ischemia of SAH patients. The predictive model could successfully predict mortality with an AUC of 0.88, the unfavorable outcome with an AUC of 0.85, and delayed cerebral ischemia with an AUC of 0.72.

SUMMARY

In conclusion, AI is a powerful tool that can be used as a useful aid for physicians. In addition, the application of AI in clinical practice requires prior knowledge of metrics and the design of models for accurate interpretation of results and model selection. These tools may contribute to the revolution of the future of medicine and clinical practice, and there is no exception for the field of vascular and interventional neurology.

DISCLOSURE

A. Mowla: Speakers Bureau/Consultant to Cerenovus, Stryker, Wallaby Medical, RapidAI, BALT USA, LLC. D.S. Liebeskind: Consultant as imaging core lab to Cerenovus, Genentech, Medtronic, Stryker, Rapid Medical. Others have no disclosure.

REFERENCES

1. Haenlein M, Kaplan A. A brief history of artificial intelligence: On the past, present, and future of artificial intelligence. Calif Manag Rev 2019;61(4):5–14.
2. Zhang C, Lu Y. Study on artificial intelligence: The state of the art and future prospects. Journal of Industrial Information Integration 2021;23:100224.
3. Buchlak QD, Esmaili N, Leveque JC, et al. Machine learning applications to clinical decision support in neurosurgery: an artificial intelligence augmented systematic review. Neurosurg Rev 2020;43(5):1235–53.
4. Kaul V, Enslin S, Gross SA. History of artificial intelligence in medicine. Gastrointest Endosc 2020;92(4):807–12.
5. Yang S, Zhu F, Ling X, et al. Intelligent health care: applications of deep learning in computational medicine. Front Genet 2021;12:607471.
6. Tangsrivimol JA, Schonfeld E, Zhang M, et al. Artificial intelligence in neurosurgery: a state-of-the-art review from past to future. Diagnostics (Basel) 2023;13(14):2429.
7. Karhade AV, Bongers MER, Groot OQ, et al. Natural language processing for automated detection of incidental durotomy. Spine J 2020;20(5):695–700.
8. Yousef R, Khan S, Gupta G, et al. U-Net-based models towards optimal MR brain image segmentation. Diagnostics (Basel) 2023;13(9):1624.
9. Abdollahifard S, Farrokhi A, Mowla A. Application of deep learning models for detection of subdural hematoma: a systematic review and meta-analysis. J Neurointerventional Surg 2022;15(10):995–1000.
10. Khalili H, Rismani M, Nematollahi MA, et al. Prognosis prediction in traumatic brain injury patients using machine learning algorithms. Sci Rep 2023;13(1):960.
11. Boaro A, Kaczmarzyk JR, Kavouridis VK, et al. Deep neural networks allow expert-level brain meningioma segmentation and present potential for improvement of clinical practice. Sci Rep 2022;12(1):15462.
12. Yin P, Wang J, Zhang C, et al. Machine learning using presentation CT perfusion imaging for predicting clinical outcomes in patients with aneurysmal subarachnoid hemorrhage. AJR Am J Roentgenol 2023;221(6):817–35.
13. Fatima N, Zheng H, Massaad E, et al. Development and validation of machine learning algorithms for predicting adverse events after surgery for lumbar degenerative spondylolisthesis. World Neurosurg 2020;140:627–41.
14. Ali S, Abuhmed T, El-Sappagh S, et al. Explainable Artificial Intelligence (XAI): What we know and what is left to attain Trustworthy Artificial Intelligence. Inf Fusion 2023;99:101805.
15. Mazzanti M, Shirka E, Gjergo H, et al. Imaging, health record, and artificial intelligence: hype or hope? current cardiology. Reports 2018;20(6):48.
16. Ursin F, Lindner F, Ropinski T, et al. Levels of explicability for medical artificial intelligence: What do we normatively need and what can we technically reach? Ethik Med 2023;35(2):173–99.
17. Yang G, Ye Q, Xia J. Unbox the black-box for the medical explainable AI via multi-modal and multi-centre data fusion: A mini-review, two showcases and beyond. Inf Fusion 2022;77:29–52.
18. Gimeno P, Mingote V, Ortega A, et al. Generalizing AUC optimization to multiclass classification for audio segmentation with limited training data. IEEE Signal Process Lett 2021;28:1135–9.
19. Erickson BJ, Kitamura F. Magician's corner: 9. performance metrics for machine learning models. Radiology: Artif Intell 2021;3(3):e200126.

20. Powers DM. Evaluation: from precision, recall and F-measure to ROC, informedness, markedness and correlation. arXiv 2020;201016061, arXiv preprint.
21. Powers DM. What the F-measure doesn't measure: features, flaws, fallacies and fixes. arXiv 2015;150306410, arXiv preprint.
22. Hand D, Christen P. A note on using the F-measure for evaluating record linkage algorithms. Stat Comput 2018;28(3):539–47.
23. Boughorbel S, Jarray F, El-Anbari M. Optimal classifier for imbalanced data using Matthews Correlation Coefficient metric. PLoS One 2017;12(6):e0177678.
24. Davis J, Goadrich M, editors. The relationship between Precision-Recall and ROC curves. Proceedings of the 23rd international conference on Machine learning; 2006.
25. Kleiman R, Page D, editors. Aucµ: a performance metric for multi-class machine learning models. International conference on machine learning. PMLR; 2019.
26. Rai A. Explainable AI: From black box to glass box. J Acad Market Sci 2020;48:137–41.
27. Needham J, Wang L. Science and civilisation in China: volume 2, history of scientific thought. Cambridge University Press; 1956.
28. TURING AMI. Computing machinery and intelligence. Mind 1950;LIX(236):433–60.
29. McCarthy J, Minsky ML, Rochester N, et al. A proposal for the dartmouth summer research project on artificial intelligence, august 31, 1955. AI Mag 2006;27(4):12.
30. Fradkov AL. Early history of machine learning. IFAC-PapersOnLine 2020;53(2):1385–90.
31. LeCun Y, Bengio Y, Hinton G. Deep learning. Nature 2015;521(7553):436–44.
32. Hwang T. Computational power and the social impact of artificial intelligence. arXiv 2018;180308971, arXiv preprint.
33. Russell SJ. Artificial intelligence a modern approach. Pearson Education, Inc.; 2010.
34. Wang F, Casalino LP, Khullar D. Deep learning in medicine—promise, progress, and challenges. JAMA Intern Med 2019;179(3):293–4.
35. Duan Y, Edwards JS, Dwivedi YK. Artificial intelligence for decision making in the era of Big Data–evolution, challenges and research agenda. Int J Inf Manag 2019;48:63–71.
36. Berry MW, Mohamed A, Yap BW. Supervised and unsupervised learning for data science. Springer; 2019.
37. Jiang T, Gradus JL, Rosellini AJ. Supervised machine learning: a brief primer. Behav Ther 2020;51(5):675–87.
38. Rosellini AJ, Liu S, Anderson GN, et al. Developing algorithms to predict adult onset internalizing disorders: an ensemble learning approach. J Psychiatr Res 2020;121:189–96.
39. Ghahramani Z. Unsupervised learning. Summer school on machine learning. Springer; 2003. p. 72–112.
40. Zhu X, Goldberg AB. Introduction to semi-supervised learning. Springer Nature; 2022.
41. Hastie T, Tibshirani R, Friedman J, et al. Unsupervised learning. The elements of statistical learning: data mining, inference, and prediction. 2009:485-585.
42. Hodeghatta UR, et al, Hodeghatta UR, Nayak U. Unsupervised machine learning. Business Analytics Using R-A Practical Approach 2017;161–86.
43. Gris KV, Coutu J-P, Gris D. Supervised and unsupervised learning technology in the study of rodent behavior. Front Behav Neurosci 2017;11:141.

44. Morid MA, Kawamoto K, Ault T, et al. Supervised learning methods for predicting healthcare costs: systematic literature review and empirical evaluation. AMIA Annu Symp Proc 2017;2017:1312–21.
45. Dineva K, Atanasova T. Systematic look at machine learning algorithms—advantages, disadvantages and practical applications. International Multidisciplinary Scientific GeoConference: SGEM 2020;20(2.1):317–24.
46. Zhang H, Zou Y, Wang H, editors. Contrastive self-supervised learning for text-independent speaker verification. ICASSP 2021 - 2021 IEEE international conference on acoustics, speech and signal processing (ICASSP); 2021.
47. Aljuaid A, Anwar M. Survey of supervised learning for medical image processing. SN Computer Science 2022;3(4):292.
48. De Sanctis R, Viganò A, Giuliani A, et al. Unsupervised versus supervised identification of prognostic factors in patients with localized retroperitoneal sarcoma: a data clustering and mahalanobis distance approach. BioMed Res Int 2018;2018:2786163.
49. Sanchez-Pinto LN, Luo Y, Churpek MM. Big data and data science in critical care. Chest 2018;154(5):1239–48.
50. Nasteski V. An overview of the supervised machine learning methods. Horizons b 2017;4:51–62.
51. Zhang Y, Wang H, Yin C, et al. Development of a prediction model for the risk of 30-day unplanned readmission in older patients with heart failure: a multicenter retrospective study. Nutr Metab Cardiovasc Dis 2023;33(10):1878–87.
52. Saravanan R, Sujatha P, editors. A state of art techniques on machine learning algorithms: a perspective of supervised learning approaches in data classification. 2018 second international conference on intelligent computing and control systems (ICICCS); 2018.
53. Sahare M, Gupta H. A review of multi-class classification for imbalanced data. Int J Adv Comput Res 2012;2(3):160.
54. Lopez C, Tucker S, Salameh T, et al. An unsupervised machine learning method for discovering patient clusters based on genetic signatures. J Biomed Inf 2018;85:30–9.
55. Alashwal H, El Halaby M, Crouse JJ, et al. The application of unsupervised clustering methods to Alzheimer's disease. Front Comput Neurosci 2019;13.
56. Panch T, Szolovits P, Atun R. Artificial intelligence, machine learning and health systems. J Glob Health 2018;8(2):020303.
57. Krogh A. What are artificial neural networks? Nat Biotechnol 2008;26(2):195–7.
58. Grossi E, Buscema M. Introduction to artificial neural networks. Eur J Gastroenterol Hepatol 2007;19(12):1046–54.
59. Renganathan V. Overview of artificial neural network models in the biomedical domain. Bratisl Lek Listy 2019;120(7):536–40.
60. Kriegeskorte N, Golan T. Neural network models and deep learning. Curr Biol 2019;29(7):R231–6.
61. Montavon G, Samek W, Müller K-R. Methods for interpreting and understanding deep neural networks. Digit Signal Process 2018;73:1–15.
62. Yu H, Yang LT, Zhang Q, et al. Convolutional neural networks for medical image analysis: state-of-the-art, comparisons, improvement and perspectives. Neurocomputing 2021;444:92–110.
63. Anwar SM, Majid M, Qayyum A, et al. Medical image analysis using convolutional neural networks: a review. J Med Syst 2018;42:1–13.
64. Markus AF, Kors JA, Rijnbeek PR. The role of explainability in creating trustworthy artificial intelligence for health care: A comprehensive survey of the

terminology, design choices, and evaluation strategies. J Biomed Inf 2021;113: 103655.

65. Guidotti R, Monreale A, Ruggieri S, et al. A survey of methods for explaining black box models. ACM Comput Surv 2018;51(5). Article 93.

66. Yu KH, Beam AL, Kohane IS. Artificial intelligence in healthcare. Nat Biomed Eng 2018;2(10):719–31.

67. Reinke A, Tizabi MD, Eisenmann M, et al. Common pitfalls and recommendations for grand challenges in medical artificial intelligence. Eur Urol Focus 2021;7(4):710–2.

68. Feng J, Phillips RV, Malenica I, et al. Clinical artificial intelligence quality improvement: towards continual monitoring and updating of AI algorithms in healthcare. NPJ Digit Med 2022;5(1):66.

69. La Cava W, Williams H, Fu W, et al. Evaluating recommender systems for AI-driven biomedical informatics. Bioinformatics 2021;37(2):250–6.

70. Johnson KW, Torres Soto J, Glicksberg BS, et al. Artificial intelligence in cardiology. J Am Coll Cardiol 2018;71(23):2668–79.

71. Miotto R, Wang F, Wang S, et al. Deep learning for healthcare: review, opportunities and challenges. Briefings Bioinf 2017;19(6):1236–46.

72. Phuong NH, Kreinovich V. Fuzzy logic and its applications in medicine. Int J Med Inf 2001;62(2):165–73.

73. Uzun Ozsahin D, Uzun B, Ozsahin I, et al. Chapter 6 - fuzzy logic in medicine. In: Zgallai W, editor. Biomedical signal processing and artificial intelligence in healthcare. Academic Press; 2020. p. 153–82.

74. Yao H, Golbus JR, Gryak J, et al. Identifying potential candidates for advanced heart failure therapies using an interpretable machine learning algorithm. J Heart Lung Transplant 2022;41(12):1781–9.

75. Chatterjee S, Das A. A novel systematic approach to diagnose brain tumor using integrated type-II fuzzy logic and ANFIS (adaptive neuro-fuzzy inference system) model. Soft Comput 2020;24(15):11731–54.

76. Sivaganesan A, Manley GT, Huang MC. Informatics for neurocritical care: challenges and opportunities. Neurocritical Care 2014;20(1):132–41.

77. Benjamin EJ, Virani SS, Callaway CW, et al, American Heart Association Council on Epidemiology and Prevention Statistics Committee and Stroke Statistics Subcommittee. Heart disease and stroke statistics—2018 update: a report from the american heart association. Circulation 2018;137(12):e67–492.

78. George MG, Fischer L, Koroshetz W, et al. CDC grand rounds: public health strategies to prevent and treat strokes. MMWR Morb Mortal Wkly Rep 2017; 66(18):479–81.

79. Liu S, Levine SR, Winn HR. Targeting ischemic penumbra: part I - from pathophysiology to therapeutic strategy. J Exp Stroke Transl Med 2010;3(1):47–55.

80. Mulder MJHL, Jansen IGH, Goldhoorn R-JB, et al, MR CLEAN Registry Investigators. Time to endovascular treatment and outcome in acute ischemic stroke. Circulation 2018;138(3):232–40.

81. Campbell BCV, De Silva DA, Macleod MR, et al. Ischaemic stroke. Nat Rev Dis Prim 2019;5(1):70.

82. Goyal M, Ospel JM, Menon B, et al. Challenging the ischemic core concept in acute ischemic stroke imaging. Stroke 2020;51(10):3147–55.

83. Subudhi A, Dash P, Mohapatra M, et al. Application of machine learning techniques for characterization of ischemic stroke with mri images: a review. Diagnostics 2022;12(10):2535.

84. Kamal H, Lopez V, Sheth SA. Machine learning in acute ischemic stroke neuro-imaging. Front Neurol 2018;9:945.
85. Wong KK, Cummock JS, Li G, et al. Automatic segmentation in acute ischemic stroke: prognostic significance of topological stroke volumes on stroke outcome. Stroke 2022;53(9):2896–905.
86. Giancardo L, Niktabe A, Ocasio L, et al. Segmentation of acute stroke infarct core using image-level labels on CT-angiography. Neuroimage Clin 2023;37: 103362.
87. Zeng M, Oakden-Rayner L, Bird A, et al. Pre-thrombectomy prognostic prediction of large-vessel ischemic stroke using machine learning: A systematic review and meta-analysis. Front Neurol 2022;13:945813.
88. Wang X, Fan Y, Zhang N, et al. Performance of machine learning for tissue outcome prediction in acute ischemic stroke: a systematic review and meta-analysis. Front Neurol 2022;13:910259.
89. Rymer MM. Hemorrhagic stroke: intracerebral hemorrhage. Mo Med 2011; 108(1):50–4.
90. Martin CO, Rymer MM. Hemorrhagic stroke: aneurysmal subarachnoid hemorrhage. Mo Med 2011;108(2):124–7.
91. Yun TJ, Choi JW, Han M, et al. Deep learning based automatic detection algorithm for acute intracranial haemorrhage: a pivotal randomized clinical trial. npj Digital Medicine 2023;6(1):61.
92. Teng L, Ren Q, Zhang P, et al. Artificial intelligence can effectively predict early hematoma expansion of intracerebral hemorrhage analyzing noncontrast computed tomography image. Front Aging Neurosci 2021;13:632138.
93. Cortés-Ferre L, Gutiérrez-Naranjo MA, Egea-Guerrero JJ, et al. Deep learning applied to intracranial hemorrhage detection. Journal of Imaging 2023;9(2):37.
94. Tanioka S, Yago T, Tanaka K, et al. Machine learning prediction of hematoma expansion in acute intracerebral hemorrhage. Sci Rep 2022;12(1):12452.
95. Pérez Del Barrio A, Esteve Domínguez AS, Menéndez Fernández-Miranda P, et al. A deep learning model for prognosis prediction after intracranial hemorrhage. J Neuroimaging 2023;33(2):218–26.
96. Rusche T, Wasserthal J, Breit H-C, et al. Machine learning for onset prediction of patients with intracerebral hemorrhage. J Clin Med 2023;12(7):2631.
97. Zhang G, Chen K, Xu S, et al. Lesion synthesis to improve intracranial hemorrhage detection and classification for CT images. Comput Med Imag Graph 2021;90:101929.
98. Ou Y, Dong J, Wu L, et al. A comparative study of chronic subdural hematoma in three age ranges: Below 40 years, 41–79 years, and 80 years and older. Clin Neurol Neurosurg 2019;178:63–9.
99. Rauhala M, Helén P, Huhtala H, et al. Chronic subdural hematoma—incidence, complications, and financial impact. Acta Neurochirurgica 2020;162(9): 2033–43.
100. Feghali J, Yang W, Huang J. Updates in chronic subdural hematoma: epidemiology, etiology, pathogenesis, treatment, and outcome. World Neurosurgery 2020;141:339–45.
101. Kwon SM, Lee MH, Seo Y, et al. A radiological assessment of chronic subdural hematomas. Korean J Neurotrauma 2022;18(1):12–21.
102. Kutty RK, Leela SK, Sreemathyamma SB, et al. The outcome of medical management of chronic subdural hematoma with tranexamic acid – a prospective observational study. J Stroke Cerebrovasc Dis 2020;29(11):105273.

103. Mowla A, Abdollahifard S, Farrokhi A, et al. Middle meningeal artery embolization with liquid embolic agents for chronic subdural hematoma: a systematic review and meta-analysis. J Vasc Intervent Radiol 2023;34(9):1493–500.

104. Colasurdo M, Leibushor N, Robledo A, et al. Automated detection and analysis of subdural hematomas using a machine learning algorithm. J Neurosurg 2023; 138(4):1077–84.

105. Biswas S, MacArthur JI, Pandit A, et al. Predicting neurosurgical referral outcomes in patients with chronic subdural hematomas using machine learning algorithms - A multi-center feasibility study. Surg Neurol Int 2023;14:22.

106. Zanaty M, Park BJ, Seaman SC, et al. Predicting chronic subdural hematoma recurrence and stroke outcomes while withholding antiplatelet and anticoagulant agents. Front Neurol 2020;10:1401.

107. Lantigua H, Ortega-Gutierrez S, Schmidt JM, et al. Subarachnoid hemorrhage: who dies, and why? Crit Care 2015;19(1):309.

108. Savarraj JPJ, Hergenroeder GW, Zhu L, et al. Machine learning to predict delayed cerebral ischemia and outcomes in subarachnoid hemorrhage. Neurology 2021;96(4):e553–62.

109. Nishi T, Yamashiro S, Okumura S, et al. Artificial intelligence trained by deep learning can improve computed tomography diagnosis of nontraumatic subarachnoid hemorrhage by nonspecialists. Neurol Med Chir (Tokyo) 2021; 61(11):652–60.

110. Thanellas A, Peura H, Lavinto M, et al. Development and external validation of a deep learning algorithm to identify and localize subarachnoid hemorrhage on CT scans. Neurology 2023;100(12):e1257–66.

111. Kim HC, Rhim JK, Ahn JH, et al. Machine learning application for rupture risk assessment in small-sized intracranial aneurysm. J Clin Med 2019;8(5):683.

112. de Jong G, Aquarius R, Sanaan B, et al. Prediction models in aneurysmal subarachnoid hemorrhage: forecasting clinical outcome with artificial intelligence. Neurosurgery 2021;88(5):E427–34.

Cardioembolic Stroke

Margaret Y. Yu, MD[a], Fan Z. Caprio, MD[b,*],
Richard A. Bernstein, MD, PhD[b]

KEYWORDS

- Cardioembolic stroke • Ischemic stroke • Atrial fibrillation • Cardiomyopathy
- Paradoxic embolization

KEY POINTS

- The main mechanisms for cardioembolic strokes include (1) valvular disease, (2) structural heart disease, (3) dysrhythmias, and (4) paradoxic embolization.
- Evaluation for cardioembolic strokes includes cardiac imaging, cardiac monitoring, and assessment of risk factors that increase the risk for patients to have embolism from an intracardiac source.
- Treatment is dependent on determining the potential source of the embolism and using a data-driven approach to determine the best preventative strategies.

INTRODUCTION: HISTORY, DEFINITIONS AND BackgroundPrevalance AND INCIDENCE

The Trial of Org 10172 in Acute Stroke Treatment (TOAST) classification system allows for subtyping of ischemic stroke (IS) by likely etiology: (1) large artery atherosclerosis, (2) cardioembolism, (3) small vessel occlusion, (4) stroke of other determined etiology, and (5) stroke of undetermined etiology (cryptogenic). Cardioembolic stroke (CES) is defined as a cortical, cerebellar, brainstem, or subcortical infarct greater than 1.5 cm and an intracardiac/aortic source of embolism.[1] This review will be focused on intracardiac sources of embolism. High-risk sources include atrial fibrillation (AFib; and flutter), intracardiac thrombus, myocardial infarction (MI) occurring less than 4 weeks prior, mechanical prosthetic valves, endocarditis (both infectious and marantic), rheumatic heart disease, dilated cardiomyopathy, and patent foramen ovale (PFO) with thrombus in situ. CES can also be a complication of coronary procedures.[2]

The American Heart Association / American Stroke Association (AHA/ASA) 2021 guidelines for the prevention of stroke in patients with stroke and transient ischemic attack (TIA) outline a basic diagnostic evaluation that should be conducted in all patients who present with symptoms concerning for cerebral ischemia: at least 24 hours

[a] University of Illinois at Chicago, Chicago, IL, USA; [b] Northwestern University, 625 N. Michigan Avenue, Suite 1150, Chicago, IL 60611, USA
* Corresponding author.
E-mail address: fan-zhang@northwestern.edu

Neurol Clin 42 (2024) 651–661
https://doi.org/10.1016/j.ncl.2024.03.002   **neurologic.theclinics.com**
0733-8619/24/© 2024 Elsevier Inc. All rights are reserved, including those for text and data mining, AI training, and similar technologies.

of continuous electrocardiography, transthoracic echo (TTE) to look for source of embolism, assessment of intracranial and extracranial vasculature, basic laboratory values (including low-density lipoprotein cholesterol [LDL] and hemoglobin A1C test [A1C]).[3]

Embolic strokes of uncertain source (ESUS) are nonlacunar IS with an embolic-appearing pattern but no clear embolic source after initial workup. There is overlap between CES, cryptogenic strokes, and ESUS. In some patients, the initial etiology of IS was unclear but an intracardiac source is eventually found.

It is important to note that patients may have competing stroke mechanisms and multiple risk factors for IS. Clinical judgment is important in those cases.

PREVALENCE/INCIDENCE

On a yearly basis, 26 million people experience stroke in the world. Two-thirds of these strokes are ischemic. CES accounts for around 25% of all IS and tends to cause more severe injury, leading to higher subsequent disability.[2] (**Table 1**).

DISCUSSION
Atrial Fibrillation

AFib is the most common cause of CES, accounting for 25% to 30% of cases. Valvular AFib is AFib in the presence of moderate-to-severe mitral valve disease. Most thrombi arise from the left atrium and the left atrial appendage (LAA). The most sensitive imaging modality to visualize the LAA is through a transesophageal echo (TEE) because of the proximity between the transducer with the posterior aspect of the heart. TEE can visualize thrombi as small as 3 mm in diameter.[6] TEE can also measure flow velocities in the LAA and define appendage morphology. LAA emptying velocities of less than 0.2 m/s is associated with an increased risk of IS.[7]

The risk of IS due to AFib can be stratified based on validated prediction scores: Congestive heart failure, Age, Diabetes, Stroke ($CHADS_2$) and Congestive heart failure, Age, Sex, Hypertension, Stroke, Vascular disease, Diabetes (CHA_2DS_2–VASc). It is important to note that these stratification methods are only validated in AFib that is clinically apparent and detected by less sensitive methods such as biennial examinations, interim hospitalizations, sporadic electrocardiography (EKG), or short-term Holter monitoring.[10] CHA_2DS_2–VASc better identifies truly low-risk patients by being more inclusive of risk factors. Patients with a $CHADS_2 \geq 2$ are at high risk for stroke, but the CHA_2DS_2–VASc helps elucidate management of patients for whom the $CHADS_2$ is 0 to 1[11] (**Table 2**).

Detection of AFib is important in a patient with stroke as it can affect subsequent management regarding secondary stroke prevention. If there is no contraindication and the CHA_2DS_2–VASc or $CHADS_2$ score is sufficiently elevated, secondary stroke prevention is typically with oral anticoagulation (OAC). Compared to placebo, vitamin K antagonists (VKAs) led to a relative risk reduction of 64% for stroke (ischemic and hemorrhagic combined) in patients with AFib. For nonvalvular AFib, meta-analyses of more than 70,000 patients have demonstrated that the use of direct oral anticoagulants (DOACs) is either noninferior or superior to warfarin for prevention of stroke or thromboembolism with decreased risk of intracranial hemorrhage (ICH).[12] In valvular AFib, VKAs are the preferred antithrombotic of choice.[13]

Paradoxic Embolization

This occurs when there is an intracardiac defect allowing venous thromboembolism to enter the arterial circulation.

Table 1
Risk of ischemic stroke with different cardioembolic sources

	IS Risk after Diagnosis	Annual Risk of IS	Relative Risk of IS
Valve Disease	Infective endocarditis: 40% Marantic endocarditis: 33%	Rheumatic mitral valve disease: 2%–5% Mechanical valve without AC: 4% Mechanical aortic valve with AC: 0.8% Mechanical mitral valve with AC: 1.3% Bioprosthetic valves: 0.2%–0.7%	Mitral annular calcification (MAC): increase in RR of 1.24/mm, increase in thickness of MAC
Cardiac Procedures	CABG peri-op stroke risk: 1.3% TAVR peri-op stroke risk: 2.3%–5.5% SAVR per-op stroke risk: 2% PCI peri-op stroke risk: 0.2%–0.5%		
Structural Heart Disease	Acute anterior wall MI: 40% acquire LV thrombus, with a 5%–10% risk of stroke related to the LV thrombus	Nonischemic dilated cardiomyopathy • EF 29%–35%: 0.8% • EF ≤ 28%: 2.5%	
Intracardiac Tumors	Myxomas: 3%–50% risk of stroke	Fibroelastomas: 6% at 1 y and 13.5% at 5 y	
Paradoxic Embolization	VSD: 6.6 cases/10,000 patient years ASD: 31.3 cases/10,000 patient years	Risk of recurrent stroke related to PFO: 2% Risk of recurrent stroke related to pulmonary AVF: 2.6%–25%	
Dysrhythmias		AFib, incidence of stroke increases with age • Patients <65 y without cardiac disease, diabetes, and hypertension: 1.3% per 15 y • Patients ≥65 y: 3%–5%/y • Patients ≥80 y: 10%/y	AFib associated with increase in RR of 1.64 compared to those without Atrial flutter associated with increase in RR of 1.41 compared to those without atrial flutter

Abbreviations: ASD, atrial septal defect; AVF, arteriovenous fistula; EF, ejection fraction; VSD, ventricular septal defect.
Adapted from Refs.[4–9]

Table 2
Ischemic stroke risk based on CHADS$_2$ and CHA$_2$DS$_2$–VASc scores

	CHADS$_2$ (Score of 0–6)	CHA$_2$DS$_2$–VASc (Score of 0–9)
Scoring Guide	CHF (1) HTN (1) Age >75 y (1) DM (1) Stroke/TIA/thromboembolism Hx (2)	CHF (1) HTN (1) Age >75 y (2) DM (1) Stroke/TIA/thromboembolism Hx (2) Vascular disease (1) Age >65 y (1) Sex female (1)
1 y stroke rate (%)	Low-risk score 0 = 1.67%	Low-risk score 0 = 0.78%
1 y stroke rate (%)	Intermediate-risk score 1–2 = 4.75%	Intermediate-risk score 1 = 2%
1 y stroke rate (%)	High-risk score 3–6 = 12.3%	High-risk score 2–9 = 8.8%

Abbreviations: CHF, congestive heart failure; DM, diabetes mellitus; HTN, hypertension; Hx, history.
Adapted from Alshehri A. Stroke in atrial fibrillation: Review of risk stratification and preventive therapy. J Family Community Med 2019;26(2):92–97.

A PFO is present in utero because the lungs do not receive blood flow. The PFO does not close in approximately 25% of the population.[14] A meta-analysis of 23 case–control studies of young patients with IS found that when a stroke is cryptogenic, there is a strong association with the presence of a PFO, which is not seen when compared to IS arising from a known etiology. Normally, the pulmonary circulation filters out microemboli that are being formed continuously in the venous system and entering the right side of the heart. Prothrombotic and vasoactive metabolites are also typically filtered by the pulmonary arterial circulation. Different structural characteristics of the PFO can increase the risk of recurrent IS; these include (1) a large residual Eustachian valve (directs jet of blood toward the PFO); (2) presence of atrial septal aneurysm (causes turbulent blood flow in the region of the PFO increasing risk of direct thrombus formation); and (3) shunt size (larger shunts have been associated with increased risk of recurrent IS).[15] Studies have shown that in situ PFO thrombi are more commonly detected in patients with IS and migraines, compared to those who are asymptomatic. In addition, the presence of in situ thrombus is significantly associated with increased stroke risk (odds ratio [OR] of 4.59).[16]

TEE is considered the gold standard for diagnosis of a PFO, with sensitivity of 91% to 100% and accuracy of 88% to 97%.[17] TTE has lower sensitivity of 45.1%, but specificity is around 99.6%.[18] Transcranial Doppler to assess for a right-to-left shunt is also a good alternative with sensitivity of 97% and specificity of 93% when compared to TEE.[17]

Treatment of PFO requires close collaboration between a neurologist and a cardiologist. Medical management is typically with an antithrombotic. If deep venous thrombosis (DVT) is present, anticoagulation (AC) is the treatment of choice. Without the presence of a DVT, the PICSS substudy of WARSS demonstrated no benefit of warfarin compared to aspirin with either the risk of IS or death at 2 years.[19] There have been 6 RCTs that have demonstrated that percutaneous PFO closure is associated with reduced risk of recurrent events. The careful selection criteria for appropriate patients include age less than 60, higher Risk of Paradoxic Embolism (RoPE) scores, and high-risk PFO features. The RoPE score is a way to estimate the likelihood that the

PFO is causally related to the stroke. The number needed to treat is 24 to prevent 1 IS over 5 years. Closing the PFO does not protect patients against other etiologies of IS, and patients can develop postoperative AFib.[15] PFO can be difficult to distinguish from an atrial septal defect (ASD), but TEE with postprocessing is better adept at distinguishing the different morphologies.[20]

Pulmonary AV malformations (PAVMs) are rare but can also cause paradoxic embolization. It can be associated with conditions such as Morbus Osler. When the PAVM is deemed to be symptomatic and a potential etiology of IS, surgery and catheter-based approaches are typically the management of choice.[21]

Intracardiac tumors

Intracardiac tumors overall have low prevalence. Myxomas are typically found in the left atrium. They are the most common benign primary cardiac tumors. Embolic phenomenon occurs in 20% to 45% of patients. Treatment is with resection to prevent further embolization.[6]

Cardiac papillary fibroelastomas (CPFs) are the next most common benign primary cardiac tumors. It is more common in patients who have had cardiac intervention but there is at least a subset of CPFs that are primarily neoplastic in origin. The IS/TIA risk is estimated in retrospective studies to be about 6% at 1 year and 13.5% at 5 years. Thus, surgical resection as secondary prevention is the treatment of choice and commonly curative. Surgery for primary stroke prevention is not as well understood, but it can be considered when the CPF is located on the left side of the heart with high mobility.[22]

Noninfective native valve disease

Calcified aortic valve disease has been shown to be associated with IS independent of other risk factors such as AFib, but the association has not reached statistical significance. This calcified aortic valve disease is more likely a marker of increased risk, but not a direct cause of stroke. Mitral annular calcification (MAC) has been found in some studies to be statistically significant in its association of stroke while accounting for other risk factors such as AFib. Each millimeter increase in thickness of MAC has been shown to be associated with an relative risk (RR) of 1.24 for embolic IS. Both calcified aortic valve disease and MAC are associated with atherosclerotic risk factors, so prevention and treatment of those risk factors are important for both of those valvular pathologies. Initially thought to be a risk factor for stroke in the young, recent studies have demonstrated that mitral valve prolapse most likely contributes to increased stroke risk by increasing the risk of AFib and needing cardiac surgery.[5] Chronic rheumatic heart valve disease is a sequela of acute rheumatic fever (immune response due to untreated group A streptococcal infection) and affects the mitral valve typically but can also affect the aortic and tricuspid valves. Most commonly, the pathophysiology causing embolic stroke is due to mitral stenosis and/or mitral regurgitation causing progressive left atrial dilation and AFib. Independent of AFib, the atrial myopathy increases the risk of left atrial thrombus formation. AFib that is due to rheumatic mitral stenosis should be anticoagulated with VKAs.[23] Nonbacterial thrombotic endocarditis comprises sterile vegetations typically in the setting of an autoimmune disease or malignancy. Low-level evidence suggests anticoagulation with the presence of systemic embolization. If antiphospholipid antibody syndrome is found, VKAs are the anticoagulant of choice. Lambl's excrescences are tiny hypermobile strands that arise on the line of valve closure and are rarely a cause of CES.[21]

Infective endocarditis

Neurologic complications are common in infective endocarditis (IE). Acute IS manifests in about 35% of patients with IE. There is an increased risk of ICH with intravenous thrombolytic therapy used in this patient population, but mechanical thrombectomy may be a feasible option. Sixty percent of patients with IE have evidence of cerebral microbleeds on MRI, and ICH occurs in 20% of patients with IE (typically as a result of rupture of mycotic aneurysms and septic necrotic arteritis with rupture of vessel wall). As antibiotics are the mainstay of treatment, identification of the organism is a crucial part of treatment strategy; *Staphylococcus aureus* is the most frequently found organism (in ∼30% of cases of IE). Initiation of antiplatelets is not recommended as secondary stroke prevention in IE, but if there is no ICH continuation of existing antiplatelet therapy can be considered. While anticoagulation should be avoided whenever possible in patients with IE, there are some circumstances in which the anticoagulation had been initiated previously for a medical reason (such as mechanical valves or AFib). Risks and benefits of resuming anticoagulation therapy should be carefully weighed in those situations. If ICH does occur, anticoagulation should be stopped. In those patients with a mechanical valve, a multidisciplinary discussion should take place and either unfractionated or low molecular weight heparin should be reinitiated as soon as possible.[24]

Prosthetic valves

Meta-analysis of studies demonstrated that a mechanical valve faces a 4.0% annual risk of stroke, which decreased with the use of OAC to 0.8% for aortic valves and 1.3% for mitral valves. The anticoagulation of choice for mechanical valves is VKAs.[2] Bioprosthetic valves have lower risk of stroke compared to mechanical valves. Thromboembolic risk associated with bioprosthetic valves range from 0.2% to 3.3% per year, higher for mitral compared to aortic valves; stroke rates are even lower in those in normal sinus rhythm (0.2%–0.7% per year).[25] Typically, patients with bioprosthetic valves are treated with anticoagulation in the first few months after the procedure and antiplatelet afterward. TEE provides the best images of the left atrial/right atrial side of the mitral/tricuspid prosthesis.[26]

Cardiac procedures

Coronary procedures. The incidence of stroke after coronary artery bypass grafting (CABG) is 1.3%, while percutaneous coronary intervention (PCI) has an incidence between 0.2% and 0.5%. There is a higher risk of stroke in the 30 day periprocedural period with CABG, but in the post-31 days and 5 year range, there is a similar risk of stroke between these two procedures. Strokes can happen intraoperatively in CABG, due to thromboembolism (from intracardiac source, cardiopulmonary bypass source, as well as due to manipulation of the aorta) and hypoperfusion (risk factors include severe carotid artery disease and significant drops in mean arterial pressure). However, the majority of strokes related to CABG happen in the first 7 days postoperatively and is related to hemodynamic instability and arrhythmias such as postoperative atrial fibrillation (POAF). The risk of stroke for PCI is highest during the first 48 hours and is most likely secondary to dislodgement of aortic debris (including atherosclerotic disease) during the manipulation of wires and catheters. The risk for stroke is higher for PCI if specific devices such as intra-arterial balloon pumps were utilized.[8]

Valve procedures. Valve replacement typically occurs for symptomatic patients (progressive congestive heart failure, exercise intolerance, and so forth). Surgical aortic valve replacement (SAVR) involves sternotomy and open-heart surgery with cardiac bypass. Transcatheter aortic valve replacement (TAVR) is a catheter-based approach with endovascular placement of balloon-expandable devices. Initial data demonstrated higher rates of IS in TAVR compared to SAVR but subsequent data suggest similar rates of periprocedural IS (∼1%–5%).[8]

Left ventricle cardiomyopathy
The annual stroke risk in patients with cardiomyopathy is presumed to be underestimated, at around 1.3% to 3.5% per year. Lower ejection fraction (EF) leads to higher stroke risk. Thrombus formation is also more common in this population—whether it is in the setting of an acute MI typically in the anteroapical territory or due to reduced systolic function leading to increased pooling of blood.[6] There are 3 types of left ventricle (LV) thrombi: mural (flat with 1 surface exposed), protruding, and mobile. The risk of embolization depends on the mobility of the thrombi. LV aneurysm thrombi are less likely to embolize as the aneurysm does not contract. Treatment is typically with anticoagulation, often with VKA but there are emerging data that DOACs are noninferior.[7] The gold diagnostic standard is cardiac MRI, which can determine underlying causes for cardiac dysfunction and the extent of myocardial scarring/viability. TEE is not effective as the apex is often foreshortened.[27]

Anticoagulation is not recommended for primary stroke prevention with heart failure alone, but indirect evidence from Warfarin and Aspirin in Patients with Heart Failure and Sinus Rhythm (WARCEF) suggests that in patients with prior stroke and heart failure, there is a role for anticoagulation, especially with EF less than 15%.[2]

CONTROVERSIES
What Qualifies as Clinically Significant/Actionable Atrial Fibrillation When It Is Detected on Implantable Cardiac Monitors?

Stroke risk secondary to asymptomatic, device-detected AFib may not be accurately reflected by current scoring methods such as $CHADS_2$ and CHA_2DS_2–VASc scores. It is known that the more AFib is monitored for, the more AFib will be detected, regardless of stroke etiology. CRYSTAL-AF and STROKE-AF both showed around approximately 12% AFib detection rate with prolonged monitoring despite the former studying cryptogenic strokes and the latter studying strokes attributable to cervical or intracranial atherosclerosis or small vessel disease. Thus, it is possible that AFib is merely an incidental background rhythm or be a marker of overall increased IS risk. When AFib is subsequently detected on implantable cardiac monitors (ICMs), secondary stroke prevention is typically switched to AC. However, the benefit from this switch is not demonstrated. In the LOOP study, while longer cardiac monitoring had 3 times increase in detection of AFib and initiation of anticoagulation, there was no significant reduction in the risk of stroke or systemic arterial embolism.[28] A retrospective study found low annual risks of stroke and systemic embolism (SES) in nonanticoagulated AFib detected on ICM, and the risk can be further stratified by duration of AFib and CHA2DS2–VASc scores. Even in a high-risk group (CHA2DS2–VASc $\geq$5), the annual risk of systemic embolism (SES) is as follows for each maximum daily AFib burden: no AFib (1.79%), AFib 6 minutes to 23.5 hours (2.21%), and greater than 23.5 hours (1.68%). The event rate of SSE in this retrospective study was similar in the anticoagulated and nonanticoagulated populations.[29]

Thus, there are no established guidelines as to how ICM-detected AFib relates to the index stroke, how it can impact stroke recurrence, and what the optimal prevention strategy for future stroke prevention should be. Results from the Apixaban for the Reduction of Thrombo-Embolism in Patients with Device-Detected Subclinical Atrial Fibrillation (ARTESIA) and the Non-Vitamin K Antagonist Oral Anticoagulants in Patients wiht Atrial High-Rate Episodes (NOAH-AFNET 6) trials may further help clinicians tailor management.[10]

What Should Be Done for Postoperative Atrial Fibrillation?

POAF occurs in 25% to 40% of patients who undergo cardiac surgery. In one observational study, 50% of patients with POAF developed late AFib. Guidelines suggest initiating OAC if the POAF lasts more than 48 hours and the CHADS2 score is ≥ 2. Treatment duration is typically around 4 weeks after sinus rhythm is restored.[30] The increased risk of stroke with POAF for cardiac surgery is in early postoperative period.[31]

What Is the Treatment of Choice When a Patient Has a Recurrent Ischemic Stroke While on Anticoagulation for Atrial Fibrillation?

Other contributing risk factors, such as hypercoagulable state (whether from occult malignancy or presence of genetic factors such as factor V Leiden) can be assessed for.

Noncompliance and nonadherence can contribute to the etiology of recurrent cerebral ischemia, especially subtherapeutic levels if on VKA. If there is no contraindication to a DOAC and that may help with compliance, it is reasonable to switch from VKA to a DOAC.

One-fourth to one-third of IS in patients who have AFib occur while on anticoagulation. Switching between anticoagulation does not seem to decrease this risk, and these patients are at high risk for recurrent stroke events.[32]

What Is the Optimal Secondary Prevention Strategy of Ischemic Stroke in Patients with Cerebral Amyloid Angiopathy?

Cerebral amyloid angiopathy (CAA) increases the risk of ICH. However, these patients often have other factors that also increase their risk of IS—AFib, antiphospholipid syndrome (APLS), and prosthetic intracardiac valves.

Surgical occlusion of the LAA is an emerging method of secondary stroke prevention for patients with AFib who cannot tolerate long-term anticoagulation. While there are early procedure-related complications, LAA occlusion could be a feasible option when patients cannot tolerate long-term warfarin. PRAGUE-17 demonstrated that LAA occlusion is noninferior compared to DOACs with a broad composite endpoint that combined safety and efficacy events. However, LAA occlusion does not protect against the 10% of thrombi that are formed outside of the LAA.[33] (**Table 3**).

FUTURE DIRECTIONS
"Pill-in-Pocket" Anticoagulation with Atrial Fibrillation

There are some case–crossover studies that show a temporal association between multihour AFib episodes and stroke. There was an odds ratio increased risk of 3.71

Table 3
Possible management options for pathologies requiring AC in cerebral amyloid angiopathy

	Possible Strategies
Nonvalvular AFib	Consider left atrial appendage closure (needs ~45 d of antithrombotics for device endothelization), after which may not need long-term antithrombotics
APLS	Risk of arterial/venous thromboembolism so high, may need to continue AC despite risks
Mechanical intracardiac valves	Significant risk of device thrombosis, consider replacement with bioprosthetic valve
Intracardiac thrombus	May need short-term course of AC
Deep vein thrombosis, pulmonary embolism	Consider inferior vena cava filters, may need short course of anticoagulation

Adapted from Kozberg M, Perosa V, van Veluw S. A practical approach to the management of cerebral amyloid angiopathy. International Journal of Stroke 2021;16(4):356–369.

for AFib episodes greater than 5.5 hours, and the highest risk of stroke was within 5 days of the AFib episode. Photoplethysmography-based monitoring for AFib detection can be accurate with smart devices. The REACT-AF trial is starting to enroll patients and will compare chronic anticoagulation (standard of care) with smartwatch-guided notification to take an novel oral anticoagulant (NOAC) in response to a single episode of continuous AFib greater than 1 hour. Data from this trial will be looking for the primary endpoint of noninferiority (combination of stroke, arterial embolism, and all-cause mortality), and the secondary endpoint is to look for superiority for major bleeds.[34]

Are Future Trials Necessary to Better Find an Enriched Population of Patients with Embolic Strokes of Uncertain Source Who May Benefit from AC?

Epidemiologic studies have demonstrated that biomarkers suggesting atrial enlargement (eg, increased p-wave terminal force in lead V1, increased N-terminal pro-b-type natriuretic peptide) are associated with an increased risk of IS. Other markers of high risk of atrial thromboembolism include high-risk LAA morphology, reduced LAA flow velocity and LAA fibrosis.[19]

Unfortunately, currently published trials do not show how best to manage patients with ESUS with those findings. Both NAVIGATE-ESUS and RESPECT-ESUS did not find benefit in DOAC versus aspirin in recurrent stroke risk for patients with ESUS. Post hoc analysis demonstrated that markers of atrial cardiopathy may help distinguish a population of patients with ESUS who may benefit from DOAC. However, many of the markers of atrial cardiopathy are also predictors for development of AFib; it is unclear whether the benefit with AC is due to the presence of AFib. A trial conducted in patients with ESUS and objective evidence of increased cardiac thromboembolism risk to see whether apixaban would be beneficial over aspirin Apixaban versus Aspirin for Embolic Stroke of Undetermined Source (ATTICUS) was stopped early for futility.[19] Preliminary data from ARCADIA presented at the European Stroke Organisation conference in 2023 suggests that even in patients with ESUS and signs of atrial cardiopathy, apixaban is no better than aspirin in prevention of recurrent strokes. More specific biomarkers need to be identified and validated to stratify patients with ESUS to those who would be more likely to benefit from AC.

CLINICS CARE POINTS

- While CES makes up just 25% of all IS, they are associated with high morbidity and mortality given that the emboli can often get lodged in large intracranial vessels, causing large areas of cerebral ischemia.

- Once a cardioembolic etiology of the index stroke is determined, treatment options depend on the source of the cardioembolism and there are ways to individualize treatment to each patient's specific characteristics.

- There is overlap between CES, cryptogenic stroke, and ESUS. Anticoagulation is not the treatment of choice for all patients with ESUS, but there is likely a subgroup that can benefit from anticoagulation but that has not been completely elucidated yet.

- As more AFib is being detected by ICM, decisions on when to initiate anticoagulation become more nuanced as the risks associated with device-detected AFib need to be better understood.

DISCLOSURE

M.Y Yu and F.Z Caprio have no relevant disclosure. R.A. Bernstein has been a speaker and consultant for Medtronic, Astra Zeneca, Bristo Myers Squibb, Boehringer Ingelheim, and Abbott.

REFERENCES

1. Adams H, Bendixen B, Kappelle L, et al. Classification of subtype of acute ischemic stroke. Definitions for use in a multicenter clinical trial. TOAST. Trial of Org 10172 in acute stroke treatment. Stroke 1993;24(1):35–41.
2. Kamel H, Healey J. Cardioembolic stroke. Circ Res 2017;120(3):514–26.
3. Kleindorfer D, Towfighi A, Chaturvedi S, et al. 2021 guideline for the prevention of stroke in patients with stroke and transient ischemic attack: a guideline from the american heart association/american stroke association. Stroke 2021;52(7): e364–467.
4. Giang K, Fedchenko M, Dellborg M, et al. Burden of ischemic stroke in patients with congenital heart disease: a nationwide, case-control study. J Am Heart Assoc 2021;10(13):e020939.
5. Mayfield J, Otto C. Stroke and noninfective native valvular disease. Curr Cardiol Rep 2023;25(5):333–48.
6. Mikati I, Ibrahim Z. Cardioembolic stroke. In: Warlow's stroke: practical management. Hoboken: Wiley Blackwell; 2019. p. 241–66.
7. Greer D, Aparicio H, Siddiqi O, et al. Cardiac diseases. In: Stroke pathophysiology, diagnosis, and management. Philadephia: Elsevier. P.477-487.
8. Hotson J. Neurologic complications of cardiac surgery. In: Aminoff's neurology and general medicine. London: Academic Press; 2014. p. 49–63.
9. Kinsella J, Gladstone D. Neurologic manifestations of acquired cardiac disease, arrythmias, and interventional cardiology. London: Academic Press; 2014. p. 79–97.
10. Kim A, Kamel H, Bernstein R, et al. Controversies in stroke: should patients with embolic stroke of undetermined source undergo intensive heart rhythm monitoring with an implantable loop monitor? Stroke 2022;53(10):3243–7.
11. Alshehri A. Stroke in atrial fibrillation: review of risk stratification and preventive therapy. J Family Community Med 2019;26(2):92–7.
12. Botto G, Ameri P, De Caterina R. Many good reasons to switch from vitamin k antagonists to non-vitamin k antagonists in patients with non-valvular atrial fibrillation. J Clin Med 2021;10(13):2866.
13. Lip G. Anticoagulation in Atrial Fibrillation and Rheumatic Heart Disease. N Engl J Med 2022;387(11):1036–8.
14. Homma S, Sacco R. Patent foramen ovale and stroke. Circulation 2005;112(7): 1063–72.
15. Mac Grory B, Ohman E, Feng W, et al. Advances in the management of cardioembolic stroke associated with patent foramen ovale. BMJ 2022;9(376): e063161.
16. Yan C, Li H, Wang C, et al. Frequency and size of in situ thrombus within patent foramen ovale. Stroke 2023;54(5):1205–13.
17. Mojadidi M, Roberts S, Winoker J, et al. Accuracy of transcranial Doppler for the diagnosis of intracardiac right-to-left shunt: a bivariate meta-analysis of prospective studies. JACC Cardiovasc Imaging 2014;7(3):236–50.
18. Katsanos A, Psaltopoulou T, Sergentanis T, et al. Transcranial Doppler versus transthoracic echocardiography for the detection of patent foramen ovale in

patients with cryptogenic cerebral ischemia: A systematic review and diagnostic test accuracy meta-analysis. Ann Neurol 2016;79(4):625–35.

19. Yaghi S. Diagnosis and Management of Cardioembolic Stroke. Continuum 2023; 29(2):462–85.

20. Lwin M, Mano T, Li W. ASD or PFO: state-of-the-art echocardiography says it all. International Journal of Cardiology Congenital Heart Disease 2021;6:100285.

21. Aplin M, Andersen A, Brandes A, et al. Assessment of patients with a suspected cardioembolic ischemic stroke. a national consensus statement. Scand Cardiovasc J 2021;55(5):315–25.

22. Esteban-Lucia L, De la Fuente S, Kallmeyer A, et al. Cardioembolic stroke secondary to an aortic valve fibroelastoma: an increasingly recognized rare cause of stroke. Stroke 2021;52(4):e111–4.

23. Boot E, Ekker M, Putaala J, et al. Ischaemic stroke in young adults: a global perspective. J Neurol Neurosurg Psychiatry 2020;91(4):411–7.

24. Sotero F, Rosario M, Fonseca A, et al. Neurological complications of infective endocarditis. Curr Neurol Neurosci Rep 2019;19(5). https://doi.org/10.1007/s11910-019-0935-x.

25. Heras M, Chesebro J, Fuster V, et al. High risk of thromboemboli early after bioprosthetic cardiac valve replacement. J Am Coll Cardiol 1995;25:1111–9.

26. Canali E, Serani M, Tarzia P, et al. Echocardiography in cardioembolic stroke prevention. Eur Heart J Suppl 2023;25(Suppl C):C212–7.

27. Dalia T, Lahan S, Ranka S, et al. Warfarin versus direct oral anticoagulants for treating left ventricular thrombus: a systematic review and meta-analysis. Thromb J 2021;19(1):7.

28. Svendsen J, Diederichsen S, Højberg S, et al. Implantable loop recorder detection of atrial fibrillation to prevent stroke (The LOOP Study): a randomised controlled trial. Lancet 2021;398(10310):1507–16.

29. Kaplan R, Koehler J, Ziegler P, et al. Stroke risk as a function of atrial fibrillation duration and CHA2DS2-VASc score. Circulation 2019;140(20):1639–46.

30. Gaudino M, Di Franco A, Rong L, et al. Postoperative atrial fibrillation: from mechanisms to treatment. Eur Heart J 2023;44(12):1020–39.

31. AlTurki A, Marafi M, Proietti R, et al. Major adverse cardiovascular events associated with postoperative atrial fibrillation after noncardiac surgery: a systematic review and meta-analysis. Circ Arrhythm Electrophysiol 2020;13(1):e007437.

32. Seiffge D, De Marchis G, Koga M, et al. Ischemic stroke despite oral anticoagulant therapy in patients with atrial fibrillation. Ann Neurol 2020;87(5):677–87.

33. Lévy S, Steinbeck G, Santini L, et al. Management of atrial fibrillation: two decades of progress - a scientific statement from the European Cardiac Arrhythmia Society. J Interv Card Electrophysiol 2022;65(1):287–326.

34. Peigh G, Passman R. "Pill-in-Pocket" anticoagulation for stroke prevention in atrial fibrillation. J Cardiovasc Electrophysiol 2023. https://doi.org/10.1111/jce.15866.

The Spectrum of Cerebral Small Vessel Disease

Emerging Pathophysiologic Constructs and Management Strategies

Ryan T. Muir, MD[a,b,c], Eric E. Smith, MD, MPH[a,b,c],*

KEYWORDS

- Cerebral small vessel disease • Hemorrhagic stroke • Lacunes
- Cerebral microbleeds • Cerebral amyloid angiopathy • White matter hyperintensities
- Dementia • Vascular cognitive impairment

KEY POINTS

- Cerebral small vessel disease (CSVD) is very common in the aging brain.
- CSVD can cause ischemic stroke, hemorrhagic stroke, and dementia.
- Neuroimaging standards for diagnosing CSVD have been updated recently.
- The Boston criteria for cerebral amyloid angiopathy (CAA) have been revised, including the addition of new, supportive non-hemorrhagic white matter features.
- Genetic studies are identifying new loci that influence risk of CSVD, offering clues to the pathogenesis of CSVD that might lead to new treatments.

INTRODUCTION

Cerebral small vessel disease (CSVD) results in a spectrum of neurologic, behavioral, and cognitive sequelae, most commonly from white matter hyperintensities (WMH) of presumed vascular origin, lacunar stroke, and hemorrhagic stroke. Other manifestations noted on MRI include enlarged perivascular spaces (ePVS) and cerebral microbleeds.[1,2] CSVD is the cause of up to 20% of ischemic strokes, manifesting as lacunar infarcts affecting subcortical deep cerebral white matter tracts and gray matter nuclei of the basal-ganglia or thalamus. Furthermore, approximately 85% of hemorrhagic

Sources of funding-no external funding.
[a] Calgary Stroke Program, Department of Clinical Neurosciences, University of Calgary, Calgary, Alberta T2N 1N4, Canada; [b] Department of Community Health Sciences, University of Calgary, Calgary, Alberta T2N 1N4, Canada; [c] Hotchkiss Brain Institute, University of Calgary, Calgary, Alberta T2N 1N4, Canada
* Corresponding author. Hotchkiss Brain Institute, University of Calgary, Calgary, Alberta T2N 1N4, Canada.
E-mail address: eesmith@ucalgary.ca

stroke is related to CSVD with the 2 most common etiologies being hypertensive arteriopathy and cerebral amyloid angiopathy (CAA).[3] CSVD is also a key contributor to cognitive impairment–contributing to 50% of dementia globally.[4–8] Concomitant CSVD is common among other neurodegenerative causes of dementia and the presence of cerebrovascular pathology, leukoaraiosis, CAA, lacunar and cortical infarcts, do contribute to cognitive decline above neurodegenerative pathologies alone.[9,10] Overall, mixed dementias, where cerebrovascular and neurodegenerative pathologies coexist, are the most common dementias.[11]

This article provides an overview of current pathophysiologic frameworks of CSVD, reviews emerging genetic risk factors and discusses the latest advances, and future directions in the treatment and prevention of CSVD.

THE PREVALENCE OF CEREBRAL SMALL VESSEL DISEASE

The prevalence of CSVD increases dramatically with age.[12–14] A semi-systematic review tabulating the prevalence of CSVD on MRI; the general older population reported prevalence of WMHs that ranged from 65% to 96%, microbleeds from 3.1% to 15.3%, and lacunes from 8% to 31%.[13] Given that the prevalence of WMHs increases with age and are seen in over 90% of individuals over age 65,[15,16] it may be more clinically relevant to consider whether the burden of WMHs exceeds the expected age, rather than focusing on absolute grades or volumes.

Overall, CSVD is prevalent across various cohorts including healthy cohorts, participants with vascular risk factors, and those with stroke and dementia around the world[14] – a prevalence which reflects an important global health issue that is intertwined with the global burden of dementia.[8,17–21]

PATHOPHYSIOLOGY OF CEREBRAL SMALL VESSEL DISEASE

CSVD can arise from a variety of processes that damage cerebral small arterioles, venules, and capillaries.[1,22] CSVD affects the function of the neurovascular unit–an interface between cerebral small vessels, pericytes, the perivascular space, supportive glial cells, and neurons, which facilitates the transit and clearance of supportive nutrients and waste products of cerebral metabolism across the blood brain barrier (BBB).[23]

Compromised BBB integrity is proposed to be an early consequence of CSVD. A study of 80 patients with overt CSVD and 40 age and sex matched controls used dynamic-contrast-enhanced-MRI to quantify the rate and extent of BBB leakage.[24] This study noted larger leakage volumes within normal appearing white matter, white matter hyperintensities, and cortical gray matter in those with CSVD compared with controls (after adjustment for vascular risk factors and age).[24] Therefore, compromised BBB integrity could be a biomarker of an injured neurovascular unit in the setting of CSVD.[24]

The neurovasculome plays an important role in the clearance of excess fluid and waste products from the brain.[25] Compromised clearance and downstream accumulation of toxic waste products, as well as impaired delivery of supportive nutrients across the BBB, may contribute to the injury of endothelial, neuronal, and glial elements in CSVD.[1] This process may promote oxidative stress, inflammatory responses, thrombosis formation, and may compromise the extracellular matrix of the neurovascular unit.[1,26,27] Dynamic cerebral blood flow changes adapt to cerebral metabolic needs and this cerebrovascular reactivity (CVR) is impaired in CSVD.[28] With increasing severity of WMH, CVR is impaired along with venous pulsatility.[29]

CSVD may manifest in the brain as 1 or more of several different lesion types, each resulting from different pathophysiologic processes. Because the symptoms of CSVD are often insidious or non-specific, neuroimaging is usually required to make the diagnosis. Furthermore, because the vessels affected by CSVD are so small, typically less than 500-micron diameter, the vessels themselves cannot be imaged directly. Therefore, the diagnosis of CSVD relies on recognizing characteristic patterns of tissue injury.

The spectrum of visible CSVD lesions on neuroimaging and neuropathology includes WMH of presumed vascular origin, lacunes, cerebral microbleeds, primary intracerebral hemorrhages (ICHs), superficial siderosis, enlarged perivascular spaces, and cortical microinfarcts.[1,2,30] Cerebral atrophy–though not specific to CSVD–also occurs as a result of parenchymal injury from the aforementioned manifestations CSVD.[1,31]

The vascular pathology of CSVD includes arteriosclerosis, CAA, inflammatory vasculitidies, venous collagenosis, and monogenic vasculopathies.[32–39] However, arteriolosclerosis from aging and vascular risk factors (most prominently hypertension) and CAA are by far the most common. CAA is caused by the accumulation of amyloid in the vessel wall. Aside from a few rare monogenic disorders, the amyloid is comprised of amyloid-beta resulting from the aggregation of amyloid-beta peptides created by proteolytic cleavage of the amyloid precursor protein.[40] Thus, the pathophysiology of CAA overlaps with that of Alzheimer's disease (AD) and they often coexist neuropathologically, however, most patients with CAA do not have dementia because of AD and only a minority develop AD with dementia. A schematic pathophysiologic framework of cerebral small vessel disease is displayed in **Fig. 1**.

NEUROIMAGING MANIFESTATIONS

The first Standards for Reporting Vascular Changes on Neuroimaging (STRIVE) were published in 2013 and subsequently updated in 2023.[2,12] Knowledge of these standardized criteria are essential for the accurate identification and reporting of the various neuroimaging manifestations of CSVD.[2] According to STRIVE, MRI lesions related to CSVD include: recent small subcortical infarcts, lacunes, WMHs of presumed vascular origin, perivascular spaces, cerebral microbleeds, cortical superficial siderosis, and cortical cerebral microinfarcts.[2] These are depicted in **Fig. 2**.

Recent small subcortical infarcts manifest as less than or equal to 20 mm diameter lesions with restricted diffusion restriction on diffusion weighted imaging MRI (DWI-MRI), while lacunes are established small infarcts (3–15 mm diameter) which do not exhibit restricted diffusion and have a central cavity that is T1 hypodense.[2] WMHs exhibit hyperintensity on T2-weighted sequences, affecting the cerebral white matter in deep and periventricular regions.[2] Cortical cerebral microinfarcts are small (<4 mm) strictly cortical lesions that are T2 hyperintense, T1-hypodense which can occur with or without restricted diffusion on DWI.[2]

Perivascular spaces are small (generally ≤2 mm diameter) fluid filled round, ovoid, or linear spaces with MRI signal similar to cerebrospinal fliud (CSF) (T2 hyperintense, T1 hypointense, and FLAIR isointense) (**Fig. 3**).[2] Perivascular spaces surround and follow the course of small perforating vessels in the white matter or deep subcortical gray matter structures.[2] The STRIVE criteria also include cerebral atrophy as a metric of CSVD.[2]

To detect the hemorrhagic manifestations of CSVD, T2*-weighted sequences (gradient recalled echo [GRE] or susceptibility weighted imaging [SWI]) are necessary. On T2*-weighted MRI, hemosiderin adopts a hypodense blooming signal intensity

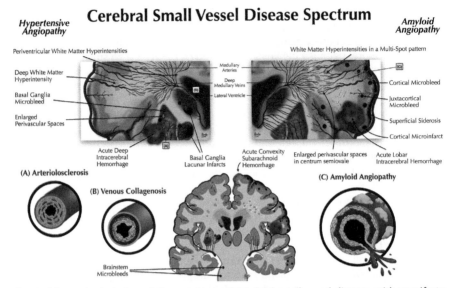

Cerebral Small Vessel Disease Spectrum

Hypertensive Angiopathy

Amyloid Angiopathy

Periventricular White Matter Hyperintensities

White Matter Hyperintensities in a Multi-Spot pattern

Deep White Matter Hyperintensity

Basal Ganglia Microbleed

Enlarged Perivascular Spaces

Medullary Arteries

Deep Medullary Veins

Lateral Ventricle

Cortical Microbleed

Juxtacortical Microbleed

Superficial Siderosis

Cortical Microinfarct

Acute Deep Intracerebral Hemorrhage

Basal Ganglia Lacunar Infarcts

Acute Convexity Subarachnoid Hemorrhage

Enlarged perivascular spaces in centrum semiovale

Acute Lobar Intracerebral Hemorrhage

(A) Arteriolosclerosis

(B) Venous Collagenosis

(C) Amyloid Angiopathy

Brainstem Microbleeds

Fig. 1. Schematic depiction of the spectrum of cerebral small vessel disease, with manifestations of hypretensive angiopathy on the left and cerebral amyloid angiopathy (CAA) on the right. In both angiopathies, cerebral white matter is vulnerable to the effects of hypoperfusion and ischemia, probably due to low collateral blood supply.[33-35] Venous collagenosis may also contribute to white matter hyperintensity (WMH) formation by causing ischemia or edema from impaired interstitial clearance.[143-145] In hypertensive angiopathy, lacunes, microbleeds, hematomas, and enlarged perivascular spaces often occur in the basal ganglia or brainstem where pulse pressure is high, but can also occur elsewhere in the brain. In CAA, microbleeeds, hematomas, superficial siderosis, microinfarcts and enlarged perivascular spaces tend to occur in the cerebral cortex or subcortical white matter, reflecting the distribution of vascular amyloid which is predominantly in cortical and leptomengial arteries and arterioles.[146-159]

(**Fig. 4**).[2] In the case of cerebral microbleeds, these appear as small ($\leq$10 mm) circular lesions.[2] Microbleeds can be difficult to discern from adjacent small leptomeningeal and cerebral blood vessels, though the key differentiating features are both size and shape (microbleeds are spherical, not cylindrical).[2] The location of microbleeds can provide clues as to the cause. Microbleeds from hypertensive arteriopathy can appear anywhere in the brain, while those from CAA tend to occur in superficial (also termed lobar) locations, because CAA predominantly affects the superficial arteries of the cerebral cortex and leptomeninges, mostly sparing the arteries supplying deep hemishperic regions (such as the basal gangalia and brain stem). The presence of microbleeds in both lobar and deep locations (**Fig. 5**) is consistent with either severe hypertenstive arteriopathy or a combination of hypertensive arteriopathy and CAA.[41,42]

Hemorrhage sensitive sequences can also detect superficial siderosis, which occurs when chronic blood products deposit over the cerebral cortex, following the undulating course of the sulci. On T2*-weighted MRI, superficial siderosis appears as a linear hypodense blooming signal over the cortex.[2] Superficial siderosis has many causes including remote subarachnoid hemorrhage, trauma, hemorrhagic transformation of ischemic stroke, cortical hemorrhage from vascular malformations or tumors, and can also be seen remotely after neurosurgical procedures.[2] In the absence of secondary causes, with increasing age the most common etiology of superficial siderosis is

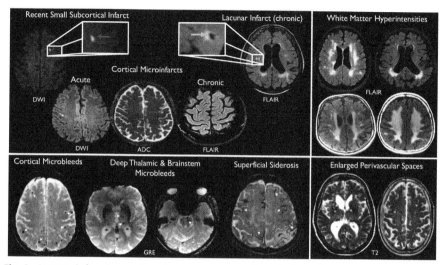

Fig. 2. STRIVE defined neuroimaging appearances of cerebral small vessel disease. There is a broad spectrum of MRI manifestations of cerebral small vessel disease. Top Left. Infarcts related to cerebral small vessel disease can appear as: (i) recent small subcortical infarcts (*red arrow*) noted on diffusion weighted imaging (DWI) (ii) cortical microinfarcts (*arrow*) which can be either *acute* or *chronic* (acute infarcts exhibit restricted diffusion (they are hyperintense on DWI and hypodense on apparent diffusion coefficient sequences); while the chronic cortical microinfarcts do not, and finally (iii) lacunar infarcts which appear as deep lesions with a central fluid filled cavity that is isointense to cerebrospinal fluid (*yellow arrow*), and can have a surrounding T2-FLAIR hyperintensity. Top Right. White matter hyperintensities of presumed vascular origin on FLAIR sequence, ranging from single punctate lesions to completely confluent lesions in deep and periventricular regions. Bottom Left. Gradient recalled echo (GRE) MRI depicting small circular blooming foci of cortical (lobar) cerebral microbleeds, deep thalamic and brainstem microbleeds (*arrows*), as well as superficial siderosis (*arrows*). Bottom Right. T2 weighted MRI depicting (*left*) enlarged perivascular spaces in the basal ganglia and thalamus (*arrowheads*) and (*right*) enlarged perivascular spaces in the centrum semiovale (*orange arrows*). The enlarged perivascular spaces appear as small, T2 hyperintense fluid filled spaces, which follow the course of small vessels and in some slices they can appear linear.

CAA injuring and promoting bleeding episodes (manifesting usually as convexity subarachnoid hemorrhage) from amyloid laden cortical and leptomeningeal vessels.[2,43]

CLINICAL MANIFESTATIONS
Lacunar Stroke Syndromes

While more than 20 lacunar syndromes were described by C. Miller Fisher, there are 5 classic and common lacunar syndromes including pure motor hemiparesis, ataxic hemi-paresis, dysarthria-clumsy hand, as well as pure sensory and sensorimotor strokes.[44] These lacunar stroke syndromes lack cortical signs (neglect, apraxia, visual field defects, or aphasia), which are often present with large artery strokes.[45] However, dominant thalamic lacunar infarcts can manifest with *cortical signs* such as aphasia[46], as well as cognitive impairment or dementia–especially those lesions affecting the anterior-medial thalamus.[47,48] Lacunar strokes can also have a variable clinical course after onset, as they are the most common acute stroke type to have a *stuttering* and progressive clinical course.[45,49]

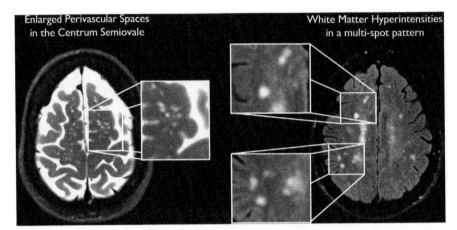

Fig. 3. Non-hemorrhagic white matter manifestations of cerebral amyloid angiopathy. Non-hemorrhagic white matter features include (1) (*Left*) enlarged perivascular spaces in the white matter of the centrum semiovale on a T2-Weighted MRI sequence (>20 visible lesions) and (2) (*Right*) white matter hyperintensities in a multi-spot pattern (>10 hyperintense lesions on MRI in the subcortical white matter on a Fluid Attenuated Inversion Recovery (FLAIR) sequence.

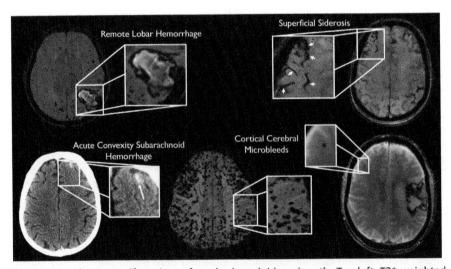

Fig. 4. Hemorrhagic manifestations of cerebral amyloid angiopathy. Top left: T2*-weighted MRI depicting a remote lobar intracerebral hemorrhage with multiple scattered cortical cerebral microbleeds. Bottom Left: Computed Tomography image demonstrating an acute convexity subarachnoid hemorrhage. Bottom Middle: T2*-weighted MRI demonstrating innumerable cortical cerebral microbleeds. Bottom Right: T2*-weighted MRI depicting a single cortical microbleed and a large left remote intracerebral hemorrhage in the left hemisphere. Top Right: T2*-weighted MRI demonstrating cortical superficial siderosis (*arrows*) in the right frontal lobe. There are also other areas in the left frontal and parietal regions with superficial siderosis as well.

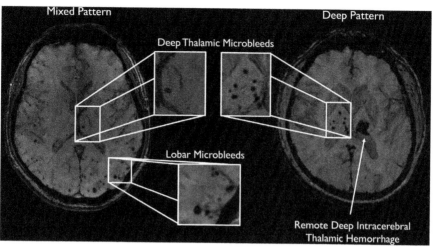

Fig. 5. A mixed pattern of cerebral microbleeds. In cases where there are both cortical (lobar) cerebral microbleeds and deep cerebral microbleeds, it is not possible to definitively diagnose probable or possible cerebral amyloid angiopath (CAA). In these mixed cases it is likely that either one of or both of hypertension and/or CAA may be contributory. The gradient echo MRI sequence on the left displays a mixed pattern, while the image on the right depicts a typical deep pattern of cerebral micro- and macro-hemorrhages (depicting multiple right thalamic microbleeds and a remote left thalamic hemorrhage).

Vascular Cognitive Impairment

Cognitive impairment is common after stroke.[4–7] Vascular cognitive impairment (VCI) refers to the spectrum of cognitive impairment following cerebrovascular injury ranging from subjective cognitive concerns to dementia.[4] Overall, both ischemic (HR=1.71 [95% CI: 1.32, 2.21]) and hemorrhagic (HR=2.59 [95% CI: 1.60, 4.19]) stroke heighten the risk of incident dementia, a risk that is modified by stroke severity, age, years of education, preceding cognitive impairment, and prior stroke.[50] While the standardized incidence of dementia 1 year following stroke ranges from 3.5% to 47.3%, depending on initial stroke severity, cumulative incidence continues to rise over the subsequent years reaching as high as 81.5% in those with severe stroke.[50] MRI measures obtained within 1 month of an acute ischemic stroke that predicted post-stroke cognitive impairment at 3 months include cerebral atrophy (OR=2.48, 95% CI: 1.15, 4.62), cerebral microbleed presence (OR=1.36, 95%CI: 1.08, 1.70), and WMHs (OR=1.26, 95% CI:1.06, 1.49), but not overall CSVD burden in fully adjusted models (OR=1.23, 95% CI:0.96, 1.57).[51]

Following lacunar stroke, the prevalence of dementia is approximately 20% and the incidence of mild cognitive impairment (MCI) or dementia is 37%.[52] The incidence and prevalence of dementia is similar for lacunar stroke and non-lacunar stroke,[52] indicating that even small lacunes can have big effects on cognition if they occur in eloquent brain regions.[47,48] The most commonly affected cognition domains in VCI are attention, speed of information processing, and executive functions such as working memory and set shifting.[4,53,54] Utilizing standardized cognitive evaluations that have been purposely designed to be sensitive and to capture the cognitive challenges faced by those with VCI is, therefore, imperative.[4]

In a large cohort of older adults without dementia, higher WMH volumes were associated with poorer memory, speed of information processing, and executive function, however, when the analysis was restricted to those with normal cognition, only WMH in occipital and temporal regions were associated with reduced cognition.[55]

Studies of ePVS and cognition have produced inconsistent results. A meta-analysis of 3575 persons from 5 studies did not note any association between global or regional ePVS counts and the Folstein Mini-Mental State Examination (MMSE) or the general fluid cognitive ability factor.[56] However, the MMSE is a crude metric of cognition. Other studies that have looked at more specific components of cognition, have noted modest associations between ePVS and cognition. In one study, ePVS in the basal ganglia were associated with worse executive function–but this association did not persist when accounting for the effect of lacunar infarcts or periventricular WMH.[57] In contrast, in a prospective cohort of participants without dementia or stroke from the Vanderbelt Memory & Aging Project, ePVS were not associated with episodic memory or language tasks, but were associated with speed of processing and executive functions and in a combined model with other metrics of CSVD, the association between ePVS and executive function and speed of processing persisted.[58] This study also found an association between cerebral microbleeds and lacunar infarcts and executive function.[58]

Greater years of education, physical activity, social engagement, and being in a marital partnership are factors that contribute to cognitive reserve and are hypothesized to increase cognitive resiliency in the face of cerebrovascular injury.[59] In one study of 10,916 participants of mean age 58.8, vascular brain injury (defined as a greater burden of WMH and non-lacunar infarcts), was associated with lower cognition as measured on the Montreal Cognitive Assessment (MoCA) and the Digit Symbol Coding Test (DSST).[59] In this study, greater cognitive reserve was indeed associated with better performance on the MoCA and DSST, however, increased cognitive reserve did not modify the association between vascular brain injury and cognitive impairment.[59] Other studies, though, have observed an attenuation of the association of WMH and cognitive impairment by increased cognitive reserve, though reported mostly for those with greater years of education.[60,61] Overall, while promoting cognitive reserve may improve cognition, this may or may not attenuate the impact of vascular brain injury on cognition and, thus, highlights the need for therapies which directly prevent or mitigate vascular brain injury.[59]

Clinical Manifestations of Cerebral Amyloid Angiopathy

The Boston Criteria 2.0, which provide criteria for definitive, probable, and possible CAA, are summarized in **Table 1**. The most notable updates to the criteria include a minimum age of 50 and the addition of 2 non-hemorrhagic manifestations involving the cerebral white matter: ePVS in the CSO and WMH in a multi-spot pattern (**Fig. 3**).[3] In addition to the neuroimaging criteria, there are 3 potential clinical manifestations out of which at least 1 must be present: (i) clinical manifestations of spontaneous ICH; (ii) transient focal neurologic episodes (TFNEs); or (iii) cognitive impairment or dementia.[3]

Boston Criteria 2.0 classify probable or possible CAA from no CAA with a sensitivity of 91.8% (95%CI: 87.6, 94.9) and specificity of 62.2% (95%CI: 51.9, 71.8) and a diagnosis of probable CAA from no CAA with a sensitivity of 79.8% (95%CI: 74.2, 84.7) and specificity of 84.7% (95%CI: 76.0, 91.2).[3]

Given that cerebral amyloid deposition occurs in cortical and leptomeningeal small vessels, CAA is associated with spontaneous intracerebral lobar hemorrhage and convexity subarachnoid hemorrhage.[3] Following a spontaneous ICH, the presence of disseminated superficial siderosis, cortical atrophy, more than 5 cerebral microbleeds, and increasing age were associated with an increased risk of new-onset

Table 1
Summary Boston criteria 2.0 for diagnosis of cerebral amyloid angiopathy

CAA Category	Criteria
Definite CAA	A. Clinical components: the patient has cognitive impairment or dementia; TFNEs; convexity SAH or primary lobar ICH B. Post-mortem neuropathology reveals severe amyloid angiopathy and no other causative lesion.
Probable CAA with supportive pathology	C. Clinical components: the patient has cognitive impairment or dementia; TFNEs; convexity SAH; or primary lobar ICH A. Neuropathologic tissue from a biopsy or surgically managed hematoma reveals CAA, in the absence of another causative lesion.
Probable CAA	A. Age ≥50 years B. One of the follow clinical features: 　i. Spontaneous ICH (brain hemorrhage) 　ii. TFNEs 　iii. Cognitive impairment or dementia C. One of the following neuroimaging features: 　i. Two strictly lobar hemorrhagic lesions on T2*-weighted MRI including: intracerebral hemorrhage, cerebral microbleeds, convexity subarachnoid hemorrhage, or cortical superficial siderosis on SWI or GRE (**Fig. 4**) 　ii. One hemorrhagic feature above with one additional neuroimaging feature in the cerebral white matter on MRI including either: 　　i. Enlarged perivascular spaces in the centrum semi-ovale on T2 or 　　ii. White matter hyperintensities in a multi-spot pattern on FLAIR (see **Fig. 3**). D. Absence of: 　i. Deep cerebral microbleeds or ICH (**Fig. 5** for example) 　ii. Absence of another cause of brain hemorrhage, microbleeds or siderosis E. Note: *Cerebellar* microbleeds, siderosis, or ICH are neither considered as deep or lobar hemorrhagic lesions
Possible CAA	A. Age ≥50 years B. One of the follow clinical features: 　i. Spontaneous ICH (brain hemorrhage) 　ii. TFNEs 　iii. Cognitive impairment or dementia C. One of the following neuroimaging features: 　i. One strictly lobar hemorrhagic lesion including: intracerebral hemorrhage, cerebral microbleeds, convexity subarachnoid hemorrhage, or cortical superficial siderosis on GRE or SWI (**Fig. 4**) 　ii. One neuroimaging feature in the cerebral white matter on MRI: 　　i. Severely enlarged perivascular spaces in the centrum semi-ovale on T2 or 　　ii. White matter hyperintensities in a multi-spot pattern on FLAIR (**Fig. 3**).

(*continued on next page*)

Table 1 (continued)	
CAA Category	Criteria

	D. Absence of:
	   iii. Deep cerebral microbleeds or ICH (**Fig. 5** for example)
	   iv. Absence of another cause of brain hemorrhage, microbleeds, or siderosis
	E. Note: *Cerebellar* microbleeds, siderosis, or ICH are neither considered as deep or lobar hemorrhagic lesions

Abbreviations: FLAIR, fluid attenuated inversion recovery; GRE, gradient echo MRI; ICH, intracerebral hemorrhage; MRI, magnetic resonance imaging; SAH, subarachnoid hemorrhage; SWI, susceptibility weighted imaging; TFNEs, transient focal neurologic episodes.

Adapted from Charidimou A, Boulouis G, Frosch MP, et al. The Boston criteria version 2.0 for cerebral amyloid angiopathy: a multicentre, retrospective, MRI–neuropathology diagnostic accuracy study. *The Lancet Neurology.* 2022;21(8):714-725. https://doi.org/10.1016/s1474-4422(22)00208-3.

dementia.[62] Furthermore, among those who survive an initial ICH, the risk of recurrent ICH depends on whether ICH is CAA related or non-CAA related.[63] CAA-related ICH has a recurrence rate of 7.4% (95%CI: 3.2,12.6) per year whereas non-CAA related ICH had an estimated recurrence rate of 1.1% (95% CI: 0.5, 1.7) per year.[63] Patients with CAA with more lobar microbleeds (>2) had a 3 to 4 times greater odds of recurrent ICH compared with those without.[63] In a meta-analysis of 6 cohorts with symptomatic ICH, the prevalence of superficial siderosis was 34% and the presence of any siderosis was independently associated with an increased risk for future ICH (HR=2.14, 95% CI: 1.19, 3.85), with disseminated siderosis bestowing the highest risk (HR=4.28, 95% CI: 2.91, 6.30).[64] In one study, patients with ICH who meet Boston criteria 2.0 for probable CAA based on two or more hemorrhagic lesions had a higher risk of recurrent ICH than patients who met criteria for probable CAA based on only one hemorrhage and one white matter feature.[65]

As CAA causes more than 50% of lobar ICH and has implications for prognosis (ICH recurrence and dementia), making an accurate diagnosis is important. When lobar bleeds are accompanied by deep cerebral microbleeds and macro-hemorrhages, it is currently not possible to discriminate CAA with hypertensive arteriopathy from hypertensive arteriopathy alone (**Fig. 5**).[3] Thus, there is still a need to improve diagnostic specificity–a potential future avenues to explore is whether fluid biomarkers of beta-amyloid may augment CAA diagnostics as they have for AD.[66]

Another clinical manifestation of CAA is the TFNE, sometimes referred to as an *amyloid spell,* which occurs in 14% of patients with CAA.[67–69] TFNEs are recurrent, transient (<30 minutes), unilateral and stereotyped motor, sensory, or visual disturbances.[67–69] About half of the TFNEs present with negative symptoms such as hemiparesis and the remaining involve positive phenomena such as paresthesias.[68,69] TFNEs are thought to be a manifestation of hyper-excitable cortex (most probably because of cortical-spreading depression, but focal epileptiform activity has also been hypothesized) that arises because of foci of subarachnoid hemorrhage, siderosis, or cortical microhemorrhage.[2,67,69,70] TFNEs may be hard to distinguish from transient ischemic attacks (TIAs). Clinicians should be aware that TFNEs can be an alternative diagnosis to TIA, because antithrombotics should be avoided in patients with CAA.[71]

Patients with CAA are also at risk for seizures. A recent cohort study with median follow-up of 35.7 months, noted that 19.7% of patients with CAA had seizures, and in 37.5%, seizures were the index clinical event leading to a diagnosis of CAA.[72] After adjusting for age and sex, the investigators found that lobar ICH and siderosis were associated with higher odds of incident seizures.[72]

The cognitive sequelae of CAA mainly manifest in the form of deficits in speed of perceptual information processing and to a lesser extent episodic memory.[73] This is in contrast to AD, where episodic memory impairment is the dominant cognitive profile.[73] In a recent study, compared with normal controls, those with CAA had lower scores in domains of memory, executive function, and speed of processing.[74] While impaired white matter integrity (measured by peak width of skeletonized mean diffusivity [PSMD] on MRI) and reduced cerebrovascular reactivity mediated the association between CAA and lower processing speed and memory, white matter integrity (PSMD), and cortical thickness in AD regions of interest mediated the association with executive function.[74] Those with the cognitive onset of CAA, compared with the hemorrhagic onset, differ also in that they tended to have greater WMH, and cortical cerebral microbleed burdens in temporal and parietal regions.[75]

Rarely, vascular amyloid in CAA can induce an antibody mediated response targeting cerebral blood vessels and resulting in cerebral amyloid angiopathy related inflammation (CAARI).[76–79] CAARI has a broad clinical presentation including acute to subacute cognitive decline (in 70%), encephalopathy (in 54%), headache (in 31%), focal neurologic deficits (in 55%), and seizures (in 37%) arising as a consequence of autoimmune related perivascular inflammation or vasculitis.[76–79]

Other Emerging and Underappreciated Clinical Manifestations of Cerebral Small Vessel Disease

Those with CSVD may also have other clinical manifestations including neuropsychiatric symptoms (eg, apathy and depression), gait and balance difficulties, and vascular parkinsonism.[80–86]

RISK FACTORS FOR CEREBRAL SMALL VESSEL DISEASE
Vascular Risk Factors

In post-mortem imaging–neuropathologic association studies, the most frequently identified risk factors for CSVD include hypertension, ischemic heart disease, diabetes mellitus, dyslipidemia, smoking, atherosclerosis, and peripheral vascular disease.[30] A pooled meta-analysis of 16587 participants across 29 studies revealed that the odds of lacunar infarction was increased with hypertension (OR=3.16, 95% CI: 2.22,4.49), diabetes (OR=2.15, 95% CI: 1.59, 2.90), dyslipidemia (OR=1.64, 95% CI: 1.11, 2.40), and smoking (OR=1.47, 95%CI: 1.15, 1.89).[87] This same analysis also demonstrated higher odds of WMH with hypertension (OR=3.31, 95% CI: 2.65,4.14), diabetes (OR=1.66, 95% CI: 2.65, 1.84), dyslipidemia (OR=1.88, 95%CI: 1.08, 3.25), and smoking (OR=1.48, 95%CI: 1.07, 2.04).[87]

Evidence is also emerging for the importance of circadian blood pressure variation and CSVD. During sleep there is usually greater than 10% drop in nocturnal blood pressure, and a recent meta-analysis of 3497 participants noted that those with less than 10% drop in nocturnal blood pressure (ie, those without a dip in blood pressure or those with reverse-dipping), had a greater prevalence of WMH (OR=2.00, 95%CI: 1.13,2.37).[88] Those without dipping in nocturnal blood pressure also had higher odds of covert lacunar infarction (OR=2.33, 95%CI:1.30–4.18).[88]

These data also beg the question of whether disorders of sleep may interrupt nocturnal blood pressure dipping or even promote nocturnal hypertension. The associations of nocturnal blood pressure patterns with CSVD suggest the possibility that night-time sleep disordered breathing could also play a role. Meta-analytic data have noted an association between obstructive sleep apnea (OSA), WMH[89,90] and lacunes.[91] One meta-analysis demonstrated a dose-response effect such that the higher the Apnea-Hyponea Index, the greater the odds of WMH.[91] While these associations do not imply causality, it is curious to note the convergence of evidence that (i) a loss of nocturnal blood pressure dip is associated with WMH and (ii) a common sleep disorder, OSA (which is known to be associated with nocturnal hypertension)[92] is also associated with WMH. Furthermore, considering pathophysiologic constructs of CSVD, it is also conceivable that OSA related hypoxia may promote ischemia in vulnerable regions of cerebral white matter.

In addition to circadian blood pressure patterns, higher systolic blood pressure variability has also been extensively studied in relation to markers of CSVD. In a meta-analysis pooling together 12309 unique brain scans, increased systolic blood pressure variability was associated with a higher odds of any CSVD (OR=1.27, 95% CI: 1.14, 1.42) an effect that was independent of mean systolic blood pressure.[93] An increased odds of any CSVD was also noted with greater diastolic blood pressure variability (OR=1.30, 95% CI: 1.14,1.48), again independent of mean diastolic blood pressure.[93]

Early Life Factors

Early life factors during peri-natal, neonatal, and childhood periods may influence the odds of CSVD later in life. One study pooled data across nearly 2000 participants from 4 prospective birth cohorts and evaluated the odds of CSVD, 5 to 8 decades later.[94] After adjustment for socioeconomic status and vascular risk factors, higher birthweight was associated with a reduced odds of lacunes, infarcts, and ePVSs; higher childhood IQ was associated with reduced WMH severity, fewer lacunes and infarcts and reduced total CSVD severity; and fewer years of education were associated with increased cerebral microbleeds and reduced brain volumes.[94] The effects of these very early life factors were independent of socioeconomic status and vascular risk factors, suggesting that there may be familial genetic factors that influence brain development and CSVD or that social and environmental influences in other periods (peri-natal, neonatal, and childhood) are more influential.

Genetic Etiologies

Classic monogenic causes

Much of the discussion this far has centered on the etiology of sporadic CSVD. There are many hereditary forms to consider. Several recent reviews have summarized the monogenic forms of CSVD along with their genetic localizations and clinical spectra including, but not limited to, cerebral autosomal dominant arteriopathy with subcortical infarcts and leukoencephalopathy(CADASIL; *NOTCH3* mutation, *autosomal dominant*); cathepsin-A-related arteriopathy with strokes and leukoencephalopathy (CARASIL; *HTRA1 mutation, autosomal recessive*); Fabry's disease (*GLA* mutation; *X-linked*); and autosomal dominant CSVD related to *COL4A1/A2* mutation.[95-98]

The typical *NOTCH3* mutations that cause CADASIL (the most common of the rare monogenic causes of CSVD) occur with a prevalence of 4 per 100,000.[99,100] *NOTCH3* encodes a transmembrane protein integral to cerebral small vessel health and is located on smooth muscle cells and pericytes.[99-101] The mutation in *NOTCH3* in CADASIL usually affects the extracellular component of this protein (in the 34 epidermal growth factor-like [EGF] repeat segment, which has 6 cysteine forming disulphide bonds necessary for the protein's integrity).[99-101] Alterations to cysteine residues compromise disulphide bond integrity in this extra-cellular protein component, resulting in aberrant deposition of NOTCH3 in cerebral small vessels, progressive thickening and luminal narrowing; smooth muscle cell alteration; and noted granular osmiophilic material accumulation within the vessel media extending into the adventitia.[98,101] Patients with CADASIL present with migraine headaches with aura, stroke like episodes, progressive cognitive decline, and dementia; their neuroimaging is typified by substantive subcortical WMH and lacunar infarcts in addition to confluent WMH involving anterior temporal lobes.[101]

CARASIL arises from an autosomal recessive *HTRA1* mutation. Mutations in *HTRA1* affect HtrA1 activity and interfere with signaling pathways involving TGF-β, which has an important role in endothelial functions of cerebral blood vessels, resulting in loss of vascular smooth muscle cells, reduction in the extracellular matrix, and intimal thickening and injury to the internal elastic lamina.[97] Patients with CARASIL in addition to stroke, dementia and WMHs, present with alopecia and spondylosis.[97] The *COL4A1*, and *COL4A2* genes produce 2 types of collagen IV that serve as major constituents of basement cell membranes, anchoring epithelial and endothelial cells to connective tissue in cerebral small vessels.[97] Mutations in *COL4A1/2* compromise the integrity of the extracellular matrix and contribute to cytotoxic accumulation of aberrant hetero-timers leading to cerebral small vessel injury and fragility.[97] Typically those with *COL4A1/2* related angiopathies present earlier in life with a variety of manifestations including ICH, porencephaly, dementia, and kidney disease.[97]

Monogenic Variants

Compared with CADASIL-causing pathogenic variants, there is a higher frequency (1 in 400), of cysteine-altering *NOTCH3* variants of uncertain clinical significance.[102] There is emerging evidence that these variants, previously deemed asymptomatic, may increase the risk sporadic CSVD.[99,102] The Cohorts for Heart and Aging Research in Genomic Epidemiology Consortium, in 2011, reported that, in patients with hypertension only, rare single nucleotide polymorphisms (SNPs) in *NOTCH3* were associated with higher volume of WMH, and more WMH progression over time.[102] This provides evidence for a role for *NOTCH3* SNPs in WMH pathobiology, and raises the possibility that some individuals with vascular risk factors may have differential risk depending on genetic composition.

In a United Kingdom (UK) Biobank study, 443 of 200,632 participants carrying *NOTCH3* varianthad greater WMH volumes (especially in the external capsule and anterior temporal lobe); cerebral microbleeds; and higher risk of stroke and dementia.[99] In a small cohort of patients with idiopathic Parkinson's disease, those with *NOTCH3* variants had nearly double the amount of WMHs than those without.[103] In another cohort with younger onset lacunar stroke before age 70 (the UK DNA Lacunar Stroke Study), *NOTCH3* cysteine-altering variants were among the most common noted, along with other variants in *HTRA1* and *COL4A1*.[104] Together these rare monogenic variants accounted for 1.5% of younger onset lacunar stroke in that study.[104]

Additional genetic loci associated with lacunar stroke have been identified as well, including several that are involved in vascular extracellular matrix integrity: *COL4A2, LOX, SH3PXD2A,* and *GPR126*.[39] This evidence is convergent with data from a meta-analysis of 21,500 cases and 40,600 controls demonstrating that a SNP in *COL4A1* was associated with lacunar stroke (OR=1.17, 95% CI: 1.11, 1.24) and deep ICH (OR=1.28, 95% CI:1.13,1.44), while a SNP in *HTRA1* was associated with lacunar stroke (OR=1.23, 95%CI: 1.10, 1.37).[105] It is interesting that genetic variants in other previously mentioned loci of the monogenic forms of CSVD appear to be associated with manifestations of CSVD.

Additional Genetic Loci

Furthermore, findings from genome wide association studies (GWAS) and whole-exome association studies (WEAS) have identified additional novel genetic loci that likely contribute to the risk of CSVD. *TRIM47,* was recently identified through WEAS at the chr17q25.1 locus.[106] The authors subsequently demonstrated (i) *in silico* evidence that a reduced expression of TRIM47 is associated with a higher risk of CSVD (ii) *in vitro* analyses demonstrated that downregulation of *TRIM47,* using small-interfering RNA, increased endothelial cell permeability at the BBB and (iii) that 2 middle aged participants in the UK Biobank with heterozygous loss of function of *TRIM47* had extensive CSVD.[106] This same study also found a novel CSVD locus in chr12q24.11, near *PPTC7,* responsible for encoding a mitochondrial phosphatase that has a role in generating coenzyme-Q10.[106]

There have been many GWAS collaborations, which have identified additional independent genetic loci (>50) associated with brain infarcts, lacunar stroke, ICH, WMHs, cerebral microbleeds, as well as impaired white matter integrity.[107] What's interesting is that while some of these genetic loci also have associations with vascular risk factors (especially the loci for WMH and hypertension), there are many that are not associated with vascular risk factors.[107] This complex and heterogeneous biology is further heightened when considering recent data from epigenetic associations with CSVD. In a recent epigenome-wide association study (EWAS), the association between WMH severity, and DNA methylation was investigated in 9732 participants.[108] This study noted novel associations with the extent of DNA-methylation, as well as differentially methylated regions (DMRs) and WMH burden, even after adjusting for vascular risk factors.[108] There were also shared epigenic loci between hypertension and WMHs in this study.[108] Overall multiple epigenetic factors associated with WMHs identified in this study may have important contributions to CVSD through diverse pathways related to immune function and perivascular inflammation; myelin, neuronal, astrocyte and oligodendrocyte development and maintenance; neurovascular integrity, clot formation, and angiogenesis; endothelial integrity and nitric oxide formation; tight-junction functions in the BBB; and lipid metabolomics.[108]

APOE-genotype

The presence of 1 or more *APOE* ε4 alleles is a well-established risk factor for lobar cerebral microbleeds and ICH.[109] One recent study combined data from several large cohort studies and evaluated associations between *APOE* and cerebral microbleeds and noted higher odds of strictly lobar cortical microbleeds among *APOE* ε4 positive individuals.[110] *APOE* ε2 positivity was not associated with microbleed counts in this study.[110] Other studies have additionally noted an association between *APOE* ε2 and *APOE* ε4 positivity and lobar ICH–an effect that was stronger in those with definite or probable CAA.[111] *APOE* ε4 positivity in this study also was associated with a higher odds of deep ICH too.[111]

A common denominator: neurovascular unit integrity

Overall, variants in traditional monogenic causes of CSVD, as well as novel genetic loci identified mostly through recent GWAS, WEAS and EWAS studies appear to be important contributors to CSVD through alterations in key proteins involved in the maintenance of the neurovascular unit: cerebral small vessels, endothelial cells, pericytes, mitochondria, BBB elements or extracellular matrix structure and function.[98,107,108] Thinking about strategies to improve the health and function of the neurovascular unit and its surrounding supporting structures may also help identify novel therapies and preventative strategies for CSVD.

EMERGING MANAGEMENT AND PREVENTION

Care for patients with lacunar ischemic stroke or ICH should follow established guidelines for clinical care.[112–114] However, there is uncertainty regarding how to prevent and treat progressive CSVD in the absence of stroke symptoms (also termed "covert CSVD"), and VCI due to CSVD, because there are no large clinical trials.

What Is the Role for Anti-platelet Medications in Covert Cerebral Small Vessel Disease?

An area of clinical controversy is whether to start aspirin for primary stroke prevention in patients without a history of stroke but with evidence of a lacune on brain imaging. On one hand, most lacunes are thought to be the result of brain infarction, which may be caused by small vessel thrombosis. On the other hand, some question whether all lacunes result from vascular occlusion, and recent clinical trials of aspirin for primary stroke prevention, such as the Aspirin in Reducing Events in the Elderly trial, were neutral with respect to the rate of cardiovascular disease, composite dementia, disability or death, as well as incident dementia and MCI.[115–117]

To date, there are no large clinical trials that have addressed the use of aspirin in patients with covert lacunes. Consequently, a writing group of the European Stroke Organization recommends against using aspirin.[113] The authors of this review generally follow this advice. However, in cases where there are multiple lacunes and non-stroke related CSVD symptoms, such as gait or cognitive decline, the authors would consider adding aspirin.[118] A review of vascular risk factors, including lifestyle and behavior, is warranted in all patients.

Antiplatelet and Vasoactive Drugs in Clinical Trials

Cilostazol, a phosphodiesterase III inhibitor, is a medication with antiplatelet and vasodilatory effects that has posited benefit on endothelial function.[119] Endothelial integrity is also augmented by a nitric oxide cyclic guanosine-monophosphate phosphodiesterase pathway and Isosorbide mononitrate (ISMN) is a nitric oxide donor that might support this pathway.[120]

A recent trial compared cilostazol, ISMN, and the combination of cilostazol with ISMN combined to neither treatment in patients with a history of lacunar stroke.[120] While the main outcome of The LACunar intervention-2 (LACI-2) was trial feasibility, the secondary outcome measures included death, drug adherence, tolerability, recurrent stroke, dependency, cognitive impairment, quality of life, as well as efficacy (a composite of vascular events, dependency, cognitive impairment, and death).[120] There were no safety concerns and the trial was feasible with good adherence and trial retention. In 153 participants, the combination of cilostozol with ISMN reduced the odds of the composite efficacy (secondary) outcome (adjusted HR=0.58 [95% CI: 0.36, 0.92]), dependency (adjusted OR=0.14 [95% CI: 0.03, 0.59]), and cognitive impairment (adjusted OR=0.44, [95% CI: 0.23, 0.85]), compared with no treatment.[120] There were no differences in the composite efficacy (secondary) outcome for cilostazol or ISMN individually.[120] These results suggest the possibility that combination cilostazol-IMN may prevent cognitive decline and dependency in patients with lacunar stroke, but this hypothesis needs to be confirmed in a definitive phase-III trial.

Hypertension Management

There is good evidence to support that hypertension management does have a role in reducing the risk of progression of CSVD. The Systolic Blood Pressure Intervention Trial MIND trial was a randomized control trial that compared intensive blood pressure management (systolic blood pressure <120 mm Hg) to standard management (systolic blood pressure <140 mm Hg).[121] This trial demonstrated that the intensive blood pressure arm had: (i) reduced risks of all-cause mortality and a composite outcome of myocardial infarction, stroke, heart failure or death from cardiovascular disease [121], (ii) a reduced risk of either MCI or probable dementia (HR=0.85, 95%CI: 0.74, 0.97) during a median intervention time of 3.34 years and median follow-up time of 5.11 years[122], and (iii) in an MRI sub-study, less progression in WMH volume (−0.54 mL over nearly 4 years of follow-up).[123]

In the Secondary Prevention of Small Subcortical Stroke trial participants with lacunar infarcts were randomized to intensive (<130 mm Hg systolic) versus standard (<150 mm Hg) blood pressure control arms and a reduced risk of ICH was noted (HR=0.37, 95% CI: 0.15, 0.95).[124]

In the Perindopril Protection Against Recurrent Stroke Study, treatment with perindopril reduced progression of WMH volume (1.6 mL less) but did not reduce the incidence of new silent brain infarcts.[125,126]

Currently, the American Heart Association/American Stroke Association and the Canadian Stroke Best Practice Recommendations suggest that for those with a lacunar stroke or ICH the initiation of anti-hypertensive medications should be considered to achieve a recommended systolic blood pressure target <130 mm Hg.[112,127] However, anti-hypertensive management solely for the prevention of WMH progression is not recommended in the absence of other indications.

Management of the Patient with Cerebral Amyloid Angiopathy

There are currently no disease modifying therapies for CAA. Two phase 2 trials, targeted amyloid aggregation or amyloid clearance, but were not successful.[128] Lecanemab or other anti-amyloid immunotherapies for AD should be avoided in patients with CAA, becasue the accelerated amyloid clearance along perivascular pathways heightens risk for amyloid-related imaging abnormalities with edema or hemorrhage.[129,130]

In the absence of disease modifying therapies, care of patients with CAA should focus on controlling hypertension, if it is present, and avoiding antithrombotic and anticoagulants unless absolutely necessary.

Additional Considerations and Future Directions

Whether multidomain dementia interventions reduce the risk of CSVD is not known. One multidomain interventional trial—FINGER—investigated the effects of a combined diet, exercise, cognitive training, and vascular risk optimization, but did not observe any differences in WMH progression or cortical thickness.[131] Two recent reviews have provided more information on recent and ongoing trials of interventions for CSVD. .[27,128] Guidance on managing VCI, including VCI due to CSVD, has been provided by the Canadian Conference on the Diagnosis and Treatment of Dementia.[118]

SUMMARY

Cerebral small vessel disease is common and presents with a broad spectrum of clinical, subclinical, and radiographic manifestations. CSVD is a direct contributor to the risk of stroke and dementia–which are anticipated to be substantive public and population health issues over the next several decades. To date, innovative work has further elucidated the pathobiology of cerebral small vessel disease including advances in the understanding of the stages of CAA and CAA diagnostics; emerging evidence supporting a possible role of venous collagenosis in WMHs; as well as a deeper appreciation for the vascular, early life, and novel genetic risk factors for CSVD. Recent updates to the STRIVE reporting standards for research into CSVD will facilitate globally harmonized methods of neuroimaging evaluation moving forward.

Overall, while vascular risk factors, especially hypertension, are key drivers of CVSD pathogenesis, emerging evidence from genome wide association studies and whole exome sequencing points to important roles for proteints involved in the structure and function of diverse components of the neurovascular unit. Epigenetic modifications are also likely to be influential. These emerging genetic factors may also have interactions with environmental and vascular risks. Perhaps future work will investigate whether subgroups with vascular risk factors may have varying degrees of CSVD risk or responsiveness to preventative therapies that are also dependent on genetic influences.

There is good evidence that controlling hypertension reduces the risk of lacunar ischemic stroke, hemorrhagic stroke, and cognitive impairment, and slows the progression of WMH.

As CSVD is a complex and multi-factorial entity, it is difficult to envision a *sole* disease modifying therapy, highlighting the need for future multi-modal and etiologically specific interventions. New trials are needed, whose methods should follow the best practices defined in the Framework for Clinical Trials in Cerebral Small Vessel Disease.[132] Some of the new, promising interventions include cilostazole and isosorbide mononitrate, minocycline, GLP1-RAs, and remote ischemic conditioning. [27,133–142] However, there is a need for more trials of interventions for CAA and genetic causes of CSVD.

CLINICS CARE POINTS

- Patients with suspected CSVD should ideally have MRI to delineate the full spectrum of neuroimaging manifestations, some which, such as microbleeds and perivascular spaces, are not visible on CT.

- Guidelines recommend single antiplatelet therapy to prevent recurrent lacunar ischemic stroke but there is uncertainty regarding the benefit of antiplatelet therapy for silent lacunes.

- There is good evidence that controlling hypertension reduces the risk of stroke, cognitive impairment, and the progression of white matter hyperintensities on MRI.

- Diagnosing cerebral amyloid angiopathy (CAA) is important, even though there are no disease modifying therapies, because patients with CAA have higher risk for recurrent hemorrhagic stroke and dementia, and when treated with anti-amyloid immunotherapies they have a higher risk of amyloid-related imaging abnormalities.

DISCLOSURE

Dr.R.T. Muir does not report any perceived or actual conflicts of interest. Dr.E.E. Smith has received personal consulting fees from Alnylam Pharmaceuticals and Eli Lilly, and has served on an advisory board for Eisai (unpaid).

REFERENCES

1. Wardlaw JM, Smith C, Dichgans M. Small vessel disease: mechanisms and clinical implications. Lancet Neurol 2019;18(7):684–96.

2. Duering M, Biessels GJ, Brodtmann A, et al. Neuroimaging standards for research into small vessel disease-advances since 2013. Lancet Neurol 2023; 22(7):602–18.

3. Charidimou A, Boulouis G, Frosch MP, et al. The Boston criteria version 2.0 for cerebral amyloid angiopathy: a multicentre, retrospective, MRI–neuropathology diagnostic accuracy study. Lancet Neurol 2022;21(8):714–25.

4. Hachinski V, Iadecola C, Petersen RC, et al. National institute of neurological disorders and stroke-canadian stroke network vascular cognitive impairment harmonization standards. Stroke 2006;37(9):2220–41.

5. Hachinski V, Ganten D, Lackland D, et al. Implementing the proclamation of stroke and potentially preventable dementias. Int J Stroke 2018;13(8):780–6.

6. Cerasuolo JO, Cipriano LE, Sposato LA, et al. Population-based stroke and dementia incidence trends: Age and sex variations. Alzheimers Dement 2017; 13(10):1081–8.

7. Sung PS, Lee KP, Lin PY, et al. Factors associated with cognitive outcomes after first-ever ischemic stroke: the impact of small vessel disease burden and neurodegeneration. J Alzheimers Dis 2021;83(2):569–79.

8. Collaborators GD. Global, regional, and national burden of Alzheimer's disease and other dementias, 1990-2016: a systematic analysis for the Global Burden of Disease Study 2016. Lancet Neurol 2019;18(1):88–106.

9. Boyle PA, Wang T, Yu L, et al. To what degree is late life cognitive decline driven by age-related neuropathologies? Brain 2021;144(7):2166–75.

10. Boyle PA, Yu L, Nag S, et al. Cerebral amyloid angiopathy and cognitive outcomes in community-based older person. Neurology 2015;85:1930–6.

11. Schneider JA, Arvanitakis Z, Bang W, et al. Mixed brain pathologies account for most dementia cases in community-dwelling older persons. Neurology 2007; 69(24). 2197–1204.

12. Wardlaw JM, Smith EE, Biessels GJ, et al. Neuroimaging standards for research into small vessel disease and its contribution to ageing and neurodegeneration. Lancet Neurol 2013;12(8):822–38.

13. Das AS, Regenhardt RW, Vernooij MW, et al. Asymptomatic cerebral small vessel disease: insights from population-based studies. J Stroke 2019;21(2): 121–38.

14. Lam BYK, Cai Y, Akinyemi R, et al. The global burden of cerebral small vessel disease in low- and middle-income countries: A systematic review and meta-analysis. Int J Stroke 2023;18(1):15–27.

15. Wharton SB, Simpson JE, Brayne C, et al. Age-associated white matter lesions: the MRC Cognitive Function and Ageing Study. Brain Pathol 2015;25(1):35–43.

16. Garnier-Crussard A, Bougacha S, Wirth M, et al. White matter hyperintensities across the adult lifespan: relation to age, Abeta load, and cognition. Alzheimer's Res Ther 2020;12(1):127.

17. Alzheimer Society of Canada. *The Landmark Study: navigating the path forward for dementia in Canada*. 1, 2022, Alzheimer Society of Canada, 1–60, Available at: https://alzheimer.ca/sites/default/files/documents/Landmark-Study-Report-1-Path_Alzheimer-Society-Canada.pdf (Accessed 10 March 2023).

18. Angeles RC, Berge LI, Gedde MH, et al. Which factors increase informal care hours and societal costs among caregivers of people with dementia? A systematic review of Resource Utilization in Dementia (RUD). Health Econ Rev 2021; 11(1):37.

19. Ovbiagele B, Goldstein LB, Higashida RT, et al. Forecasting the future of stroke in the United States: a policy statement from the American Heart Association and American Stroke Association. Stroke 2013;44(8):2361–75.

20. Bruck CC, Wolters FJ, Ikram MA, et al. Projections of costs and quality adjusted life years lost due to dementia from 2020 to 2050: A population-based microsimulation study. Alzheimers Dement 2023. https://doi.org/10.1002/alz.13019.

21. Xu J, Zhang Y, Qiu C, et al. Global and regional economic costs of dementia: a systematic review. Lancet 2017;390. https://doi.org/10.1016/s0140-6736(17)33185-9.

22. Wardlaw JM, Smith C, Dichgans M. Mechanisms of sporadic cerebral small vessel disease: insights from neuroimaging. Lancet Neurol 2013;12(5):483–97.

23. Black S, Iadecola C. Vascular cognitive impairment: small vessels, big toll: introduction. Stroke 2009;40(3 Suppl):S38–9.

24. Zhang C, Wong S, van de Haar H, et al. Blood-brain barrier leakage is more widespread in patients with cerebral small vessel disease. Neurology 2017;88(5):426–32.

25. Iadecola C, Smith EE, Anrather J, et al. The neurovasculome: Key roles in brain health and cognitive impairment: A Scientific Statement From the American Heart Association/American Stroke Association. Stroke 2023;54(6):e251-e71.

26. Regenhardt RW, Das AS, Lo EH, et al. Advances in understanding the pathophysiology of lacunar stroke: a review. JAMA Neurol 2018;75(10):1273–81.

27. Markus HS, de Leeuw FE. Cerebral small vessel disease: recent advances and future directions. Int J Stroke 2023;18(1):4–14.

28. Wardlaw JM, Benveniste H, Williams A. Cerebral vascular dysfunctions detected in human small vessel disease and implications for preclinical studies. Annu Rev Physiol 2022;84:409–34.

29. Blair GW, Thrippleton MJ, Shi Y, et al. Intracranial hemodynamic relationships in patients with cerebral small vessel disease. Neurology 2020;94(21):e2258–69.

30. Humphreys CA, Smith C, Wardlaw JM. Correlations in post-mortem imaging-histopathology studies of sporadic human cerebral small vessel disease: A systematic review. Neuropathol Appl Neurobiol 2021;47(7):910–30.

31. Ter Telgte A, van Leijsen EMC, Wiegertjes K, et al. Cerebral small vessel disease: from a focal to a global perspective. Nat Rev Neurol 2018;14(7):387–98.

32. Fernando MS, Simpson JE, Matthews F, et al. White matter lesions in an unselected cohort of the elderly: molecular pathology suggests origin from chronic hypoperfusion injury. Stroke 2006;37(6):1391–8.

33. Brown WR, Moody DM, Thore CR, et al. Microvascular changes in the white mater in dementia. J Neurol Sci 2009;283(1–2):28–31.

34. Nan D, Cheng Y, Feng L, et al. Potential mechanism of venous system for leukoaraiosis: from post-mortem to in vivo research. Neurodegener Dis 2019;19(3–4):101–8.

35. Moody D, Bell M, Challa V. Features of the cerebral vascular pattern that predict vulnerability to perfusion or oxygenation deficiency: an anatomic study. AJNR Am J Neuroradiol 1990;11(3):431–9.

36. Koemans EA, Chhatwal JP, van Veluw SJ, et al. Progression of cerebral amyloid angiopathy: a pathophysiological framework. Lancet Neurol 2023;22(7):632–42.

37. Keith J, Gao FQ, Noor R, et al. Collagenosis of the deep medullary veins: an underrecognized pathologic correlate of white matter hyperintensities and periventricular infarction? J Neuropathol Exp Neurol 2017;76(4):299–312.

38. Cao Y, Huang MY, Mao CH, et al. Arteriolosclerosis differs from venular collagenosis in relation to cerebrovascular parenchymal damages: an autopsy-based study. Stroke Vasc Neurol 2023;8(4):267–75.

39. Traylor M, Persyn E, Tomppo L, et al. Genetic basis of lacunar stroke: a pooled analysis of individual patient data and genome-wide association studies. Lancet Neurol 2021;20(5):351–61.

40. Greenberg SM, Bacskai BJ, Hernandez-Guillamon M, et al. Cerebral amyloid angiopathy and Alzheimer disease - one peptide, two pathways. Nat Rev Neurol 2020;16(1):30–42.

41. Pasi M, Charidimou A, Boulouis G, et al. Mixed-location cerebral hemorrhage/microbleeds: Underlying microangiopathy and recurrence risk. Neurology 2018;90(2):e119–26.

42. Jolink WMT, van Veluw SJ, Zwanenburg JJM, et al. Histopathology of cerebral microinfarcts and microbleeds in spontaneous intracerebral hemorrhage. Transl Stroke Res 2023;14(2):174–84.

43. Charidimou A, Perosa V, Frosch MP, et al. Neuropathological correlates of cortical superficial siderosis in cerebral amyloid angiopathy. Brain 2020;143(11):3343–51.

44. Fisher CM. Lacunar strokes and infarcts: a review. Neurology 1982;32(8):871–6.

45. Regenhardt RW, Das AS, Ohtomo R, et al. Pathophysiology of Lacunar Stroke: History's Mysteries and Modern Interpretations. J Stroke Cerebrovasc Dis 2019;28(8):2079–97.

46. Hyman BT, Tranel D. Hemianesthesia and aphasia. An anatomical and behavioral study. Arch Neurol 1989;46(7):816–9.

47. Swartz RH, Black SE. Anterior-medial thalamic lesions in dementia: frequent, and volume dependently associated with sudden cognitive decline. J Neurol Neurosurg Psychiatry 2006;77(12):1307–12.

48. Benisty S, Gouw AA, Porcher R, et al. Location of lacunar infarcts correlates with cognition in a sample of non-disabled subjects with age-related white-matter changes: the LADIS study. J Neurol Neurosurg Psychiatry 2009;80(5):478–83.

49. Steinke W, Ley SC. Lacunar stroke is the major cause of progressive motor deficits. Stroke 2002;33(6):1510–6.

50. Pendlebury ST, Rothwell PM, Oxford Vascular Study. Incidence and prevalence of dementia associated with transient ischaemic attack and stroke: analysis of the population-based Oxford Vascular Study. Lancet Neurol 2019;18(3):248–58.

51. Ball E, Shah M, Ross E, et al. Predictors of post-stroke cognitive impairment using acute structural MRI neuroimaging: A systematic review and meta-analysis. Int J Stroke 2023;18(5):543–54.

52. Makin SD, Turpin S, Dennis MS, et al. Cognitive impairment after lacunar stroke: systematic review and meta-analysis of incidence, prevalence and comparison with other stroke subtypes. J Neurol Neurosurg Psychiatry 2013;84(8):893–900.

53. Garrett KD, Browndyke JN, Whelihan W, et al. The neuropsychological profile of vascular cognitive impairment–no dementia: comparisons to patients at risk for cerebrovascular disease and vascular dementia. Arch Clin Neuropsychol 2004;19(6):745–57.

54. Muir RT, Lam B, Honjo K, et al. Trail making test elucidates neural substrates of specific poststroke executive dysfunctions. Stroke 2015;46(10):2755–61.

55. Membreno R, Thomas KR, Calcetas AT, et al. Regional white matter hyperintensities relate to specific cognitive abilities in older adults without dementia. Alzheimer Dis Assoc Disord Oct-Dec 01 2023;37(4):303–9.

56. Hilal S, Tan CS, Adams HHH, et al. Enlarged perivascular spaces and cognition: A meta-analysis of 5 population-based studies. Neurology 2018;91(9):e832–42.
57. Choe YM, Baek H, Choi HJ, et al. Association between enlarged perivascular spaces and cognition in a memory clinic population. Neurology 2022;99(13): e1414–21.
58. Passiak BS, Liu D, Kresge HA, et al. Perivascular spaces contribute to cognition beyond other small vessel disease markers. Neurology 2019;92(12):e1309–21.
59. Durrani R, Friedrich MG, Schulze KM, et al. Effect of cognitive reserve on the association of vascular brain injury with cognition: analysis of the PURE and CAHHM studies. Neurology 2021;97(17):e1707–16.
60. Jokinen H, Melkas S, Madureira S, et al. Cognitive reserve moderates long-term cognitive and functional outcome in cerebral small vessel disease. J Neurol Neurosurg Psychiatry 2016;87(12):1296–302.
61. Farfel JM, Nitrini R, Suemoto CK, et al. Very low levels of education and cognitive reserve: a clinicopathologic study. Neurology 2013;81(7):650–7.
62. Moulin S, Labreuche J, Bombois S, et al. Dementia risk after spontaneous intracerebral haemorrhage: a prospective cohort study. Lancet Neurol 2016;15(8): 820–9.
63. Charidimou A, Imaizumi T, Moulin S, et al. Brain hemorrhage recurrence, small vessel disease type, and cerebral microbleeds. Neurology 2017;89:820–9.
64. Charidimou A, Boulouis G, Greenberg SM, et al. Cortical superficial siderosis and bleeding risk in cerebral amyloid angiopathy: A meta-analysis. Neurology 2019;93(24):e2192–202.
65. Fandler-Hofler S, Gattringer T, Enzinger C, et al. Comparison of boston criteria v2.0/v1.5 for cerebral amyloid angiopathy to predict recurrent intracerebral hemorrhage. Stroke 2023. https://doi.org/10.1161/STROKEAHA.122.042407.
66. Muir RT, Ismail Z, Black SE, Smith EE. Comparative methods for quantifying plasma biomarkers in Alzheimer's disease: Implications for the next frontier in cerebral amyloid angiopathy diagnostics. Alzheimers Dement 2024;20(2): 1436–58.
67. Yamada M. Cerebral amyloid angiopathy: emerging concepts. J Stroke 2015; 17(1):17–30.
68. Charidimou A, Baron JC, Werring DJ. Transient focal neurological episodes, cerebral amyloid angiopathy, and intracerebral hemorrhage risk: looking beyond TIAs. Int J Stroke 2013;8(2):105–8.
69. Charidimou A, Peeters A, Fox Z, et al. Spectrum of transient focal neurological episodes in cerebral amyloid angiopathy: multicentre magnetic resonance imaging cohort study and meta-analysis. Stroke 2012;43(9):2324–30.
70. Apoil M, Cogez J, Dubuc L, et al. Focal cortical subarachnoid hemorrhage revealed by recurrent paresthesias: a clinico-radiological syndrome strongly associated with cerebral amyloid angiopathy. Cerebrovasc Dis 2013;36(2):139–44.
71. Smith EE, Charidimou A, Ayata C, et al. Cerebral amyloid angiopathy-related transient focal neurologic episodes. Neurology 2021;97(5):231–8.
72. Freund BE, Sanchez-Boluarte SS, Blackmon K, et al. Incidence and risk factors associated with seizures in cerebral amyloid angiopathy. Eur J Neurol 2023; 30(12):3682–91.
73. Arvanitakis Z, Leurgans SE, Wang Z, et al. Cerebral amyloid angiopathy pathology and cognitive domains in older persons. Ann Neurol 2011;69(2):320–7.
74. Durrani R, Wang M, Cox E, et al. Mediators of cognitive impairment in cerebral amyloid angiopathy. Int J Stroke 2023;18(1):78–84.

75. Perini G, Ramusino MC, Farina LM, et al. Cognitive versus hemorrhagic onset in cerebral amyloid angiopathy: neuroimaging features. Curr Alzheimer Res 2023; 20(4):267–76.
76. Auriel E, Charidimou A, Gurol ME, et al. Validation of clinicoradiological criteria for the diagnosis of cerebral amyloid angiopathy-related inflammation. JAMA Neurol 2016;73(2):197–202.
77. Antolini L, DiFrancesco JC, Zedde M, et al. Spontaneous ARIA-like events in cerebral amyloid angiopathy-related inflammation: a multicenter prospective longitudinal cohort study. Neurology 2021;97(18):e1809–22.
78. Piazza F, Greenberg SM, Savoiardo M, et al. Anti-amyloid beta autoantibodies in cerebral amyloid angiopathy-related inflammation: implications for amyloid-modifying therapies. Ann Neurol 2013;73(4):449–58.
79. Moussaddy A, Levy A, Strbian D, et al. Inflammatory cerebral amyloid angiopathy, amyloid-beta-related angiitis, and primary angiitis of the central nervous system: similarities and differences. Stroke 2015;46(9):e210–3.
80. Sharma B, Wang M, McCreary CR, et al. Gait and falls in cerebral small vessel disease: a systematic review and meta-analysis. Age Ageing 2023;52(3).
81. Hollocks MJ, Lawrence AJ, Brookes RL, et al. Differential relationships between apathy and depression with white matter microstructural changes and functional outcomes. Brain 2015;138(Pt 12):3803–15.
82. Jacob MA, Cai M, Bergkamp M, et al. Cerebral small vessel disease progression increases risk of incident parkinsonism. Ann Neurol 2023;93(6):1130–41.
83. Wouts L, Marijnissen RM, Oude Voshaar RC, et al. Strengths and weaknesses of the vascular apathy hypothesis: a narrative review. Am J Geriatr Psychiatry 2023;31(3):183–94.
84. Clancy U, Gilmartin D, Jochems ACC, et al. Neuropsychiatric symptoms associated with cerebral small vessel disease: a systematic review and meta-analysis. Lancet Psychiatr 2021;8(3):225–36.
85. Sharma B, Gee M, Nelles K, et al. Gait in cerebral amyloid angiopathy. J Am Heart Assoc 2022;11(19):e025886.
86. Martino D, Espay AJ, Fasano A, et al. Chapter 8.3: disorders of gait. Disorders of movement: a guide to diagnosis and treatment. Berlin, Heidelberg, New York, Dordrecht, London: Springer; 2016. p. 419–20, chap 8.3.
87. Wang Z, Chen Q, Chen J, et al. Risk factors of cerebral small vessel disease: A systematic review and meta-analysis. Medicine (Baltimore) 2021;100(51): e28229.
88. Chokesuwattanaskul A, Cheungpasitporn W, Thongprayoon C, et al. Impact of circadian blood pressure pattern on silent cerebral small vessel disease: a systematic review and meta-analysis. J Am Heart Assoc 2020;9(12):e016299.
89. Huang Y, Yang C, Yuan R, et al. Association of obstructive sleep apnea and cerebral small vessel disease: a systematic review and meta-analysis. Sleep 2020;43(4).
90. Chokesuwattanaskul A, Lertjitbanjong P, Thongprayoon C, et al. Impact of obstructive sleep apnea on silent cerebral small vessel disease: a systematic review and meta-analysis. Sleep Med 2020;68:80–8.
91. Lee G, Dharmakulaseelan L, Muir RT, et al. Obstructive sleep apnea is associated with markers of cerebral small vessel disease in a dose-response manner: A systematic review and meta-analysis. Sleep Med Rev 2023;68:101763.
92. Kario K, Hettrick DA, Prejbisz A, et al. Obstructive sleep apnea-induced neurogenic nocturnal hypertension: a potential role of renal denervation? Hypertension 2021;77(4):1047–60.

93. Tully PJ, Yano Y, Launer LJ, et al. Association between blood pressure variability and cerebral small-vessel disease: a systematic review and meta-analysis. J Am Heart Assoc 2020;9(1):e013841.
94. Backhouse EV, Shenkin SD, McIntosh AM, et al. Early life predictors of late life cerebral small vessel disease in four prospective cohort studies. Brain 2021; 144(12):3769–78.
95. Elahi FM, Wang MM, Meschia JF. Cerebral small vessel disease-related dementia: more questions than answers. Stroke 2023;54(3):648–60.
96. Manini A, Pantoni L. Genetic causes of cerebral small vessel diseases: a practical guide for neurologists. Neurology 2023;100(16):766–83.
97. Haffner C, Malik R, Dichgans M. Genetic factors in cerebral small vessel disease and their impact on stroke and dementia. J Cerebr Blood Flow Metabol 2016;36(1):158–71.
98. Debette S, Markus HS. Stroke genetics: discovery, insight into mechanisms, and clinical perspectives. Circ Res 2022;130(8):1095–111.
99. Cho BPH, Nannoni S, Harshfield EL, et al. NOTCH3 variants are more common than expected in the general population and associated with stroke and vascular dementia: an analysis of 200 000 participants. J Neurol Neurosurg Psychiatry 2021;92(7):694–701.
100. Hack RJ, Rutten JW, Person TN, et al. Cysteine-altering NOTCH3 variants are a risk factor for stroke in the elderly population. Stroke 2020;51(12):3562–9.
101. Chabriat H, Joutel A, Dichgans M, et al. Cadasil. Lancet Neurol 2009;8(7): 643–53.
102. Schmidt H, Zeginigg M, Wiltgen M, et al. Genetic variants of the NOTCH3 gene in the elderly and magnetic resonance imaging correlates of age-related cerebral small vessel disease. Brain 2011;134(Pt 11):3384–97.
103. Ramirez J, Dilliott AA, Binns MA, et al. Parkinson's Disease, NOTCH3 Genetic Variants, and White Matter Hyperintensities. Mov Disord 2020;35(11):2090–5.
104. Tan RYY, Traylor M, Megy K, et al. How common are single gene mutations as a cause for lacunar stroke? A targeted gene panel study. Neurology 2019;93(22): e2007–20.
105. Rannikmäe K, Sivakumaran V, Millar H, et al. COL4A2 is associated with lacunar ischemic stroke and deep ICH: Meta-analyses among 21,500 cases and 40,600 controls. Neurology 2017;89(17):1829–39.
106. Mishra A, Duplaa C, Vojinovic D, et al. Gene-mapping study of extremes of cerebral small vessel disease reveals TRIM47 as a strong candidate. Brain 2022; 145(6):1992–2007.
107. Bordes C, Sargurupremraj M, Mishra A, et al. Genetics of common cerebral small vessel disease. Nat Rev Neurol 2022;18(2):84–101.
108. Yang Y, Knol MJ, Wang R, et al. Epigenetic and integrative cross-omics analyses of cerebral white matter hyperintensities on MRI. Brain 2023;146(2):492–506.
109. Shams M, Shams S, Martola J, et al. MRI markers of small vessel disease and the APOE allele in cognitive impairment. Front Aging Neurosci 2022;14:897674.
110. Knol MJ, Lu D, Traylor M, et al. Association of common genetic variants with brain microbleeds: A genome-wide association study. Neurology 2020;95(24): e3331–43.
111. Biffi A, Sonni A, Anderson CD, et al. Variants at APOE influence risk of deep and lobar intracerebral hemorrhage. Ann Neurol 2010;68(6):934–43.
112. Gladstone DJ, Lindsay MP, Douketis J, et al. Canadian stroke best practice recommendations: secondary prevention of stroke update 2020. Can J Neurol Sci 2022;49(3):315–37.

113. Wardlaw JM, Debette S, Jokinen H, et al. ESO guideline on covert cerebral small vessel disease. Eur Stroke J 2021;6(2):CXI–CLXII.
114. Hou X, Cen K, Cui Y, et al. Antiplatelet therapy for secondary prevention of lacunar stroke: a systematic review and network meta-analysis. Eur J Clin Pharmacol 2023;79(1):63–70.
115. McNeil JJ, Wolfe R, Woods RL, et al. Effect of aspirin on cardiovascular events and bleeding in the healthy elderly. N Engl J Med 2018;379(16):1509–18.
116. McNeil JJ, Woods RL, Nelson MR, et al. Effect of aspirin on disability-free survival in the healthy elderly. N Engl J Med 2018;379(16):1499–508.
117. Ryan J, Storey E, Murray AM, et al. Randomized placebo-controlled trial of the effects of aspirin on dementia and cognitive decline. Neurology 2020;95(3):e320–31.
118. Smith EE, Barber P, Field TS, et al. Canadian consensus conference on diagnosis and treatment of dementia (CCCDTD)5: Guidelines for management of vascular cognitive impairment. Alzheimers Dement (N Y) 2020;6(1):e12056.
119. Ip BYM, Lam BYK, Hui VMH, et al. Efficacy and safety of cilostazol in decreasing progression of cerebral white matter hyperintensities-A randomized controlled trial. Alzheimers Dement (N Y) 2022;8(1):e12369.
120. Wardlaw JM, Woodhouse LJ, Mhlanga II, et al. Isosorbide mononitrate and cilostazol treatment in patients with symptomatic cerebral small vessel disease: the lacunar intervention trial-2 (LACI-2) randomized clinical trial. JAMA Neurol 2023;80(7):682–92.
121. Wright JT Jr, Williamson JD, Whelton PK, et al. A randomized trial of intensive versus standard blood-pressure control. N Engl J Med 2015;373(22):2103–16.
122. Williamson JD, Pajewski NM, Auchus AP, et al. Effect of intensive vs standard blood pressure control on probable dementia: a randomized clinical trial. JAMA 2019;321(6):553–61.
123. Nasrallah IM, Pajewski NM, Auchus AP, et al. Association of intensive vs standard blood pressure control with cerebral white matter lesions. JAMA 2019;322(6):524–34.
124. Study Group, Benavente OR, Coffey CS, Conwit R, et al. Blood-pressure targets in patients with recent lacunar stroke: the SPS3 randomised trial. Lancet 2013;382(9891):507–15.
125. Dufouil C, Chalmers J, Coskun O, et al. Effects of blood pressure lowering on cerebral white matter hyperintensities in patients with stroke: the PROGRESS (Perindopril Protection Against Recurrent Stroke Study) Magnetic Resonance Imaging Substudy. Circulation 2005;112(11):1644–50.
126. Hasegawa Y, Yamaguchi T, Omae T, et al. Effects of perindopril-based blood pressure lowering and of patient characteristics on the progression of silent brain infarct: the Perindopril Protection against Recurrent Stroke Study (PROGRESS) CT Substudy in Japan. Hypertens Res 2004;27(3):147–56.
127. Kleindorfer DO, Towfighi A, Chaturvedi S, et al. 2021 Guideline for the prevention of stroke in patients with stroke and transient ischemic attack: a guideline from the American heart association/American stroke association. Stroke 2021;52(7):e364–467.
128. Smith EE, Markus HS. New Treatment Approaches to Modify the Course of Cerebral Small Vessel Diseases. Stroke 2020;51(1):38–46.
129. Smith EE, Greenberg SM, Black SE. The impending era of beta-amyloid therapy: Clinical and research considerations for treating vascular contributions to neurodegeneration. Cerebral Circulation - Cognition and Behavior 2023. https://doi.org/10.1016/j.cccb.2023.100159.

130. Reish NJ, Jamshidi P, Stamm B, et al. Multiple Cerebral Hemorrhages in a Patient Receiving Lecanemab and Treated with t-PA for Stroke. N Engl J Med 2023. https://doi.org/10.1056/NEJMc2215148.

131. Stephen R, Liu Y, Ngandu T, et al. Brain volumes and cortical thickness on MRI in the Finnish Geriatric Intervention Study to Prevent Cognitive Impairment and Disability (FINGER). Alzheimer's Res Ther 2019;11(1):53.

132. Markus HS, van Der Flier WM, Smith EE, et al. Framework for Clinical Trials in Cerebral Small Vessel Disease (FINESSE): A Review. JAMA Neurol 2022; 79(11):1187–98.

133. Yan P, Zhu A, Liao F, et al. Minocycline reduces spontaneous hemorrhage in mouse models of cerebral amyloid angiopathy. Stroke 2015;46(6):1633–40.

134. Voigt S, Koemans EA, Rasing I, et al. Minocycline for sporadic and hereditary cerebral amyloid angiopathy (BATMAN): study protocol for a placebo-controlled randomized double-blind trial. Trials 2023;24(1):378.

135. Ganesh A, Barber P, Black SE, et al. Trial of remote ischaemic preconditioning in vascular cognitive impairment (TRIC-VCI): protocol. BMJ Open 2020;10(10): e040466.

136. Ballard C, Nørgaard CH, Friedrich S, et al. Liraglutide and semaglutide: Pooled post hoc analysis to evaluate risk of dementia in patients with type 2 diabetes. Alzheimer's Dementia 2020;16(S9).

137. Cukierman-Yaffe T, Gerstein HC, Colhoun HM, et al. Effect of dulaglutide on cognitive impairment in type 2 diabetes: an exploratory analysis of the REWIND trial. Lancet Neurol 2020;19(7):582–90.

138. Norgaard CH, Friedrich S, Hansen CT, et al. Treatment with glucagon-like peptide-1 receptor agonists and incidence of dementia: Data from pooled double-blind randomized controlled trials and nationwide disease and prescription registers. Alzheimers Dement (N Y) 2022;8(1):e12268.

139. Dei Cas A. Long-acting exenatide and cognitive decline in dysglycemic patients (DRINN). clinicaltrials.gov. Available at: https://www.clinicaltrials.gov/ct2/show/NCT02847403. [Accessed 29 March 2023].

140. Bellastella G, Maiorino MI, Longo M, et al. Glucagon-like peptide-1 receptor agonists and prevention of stroke systematic review of cardiovascular outcome trials with meta-analysis. Stroke 2020;51(2):666–9.

141. Femminella GD, Frangou E, Love SB, et al. Evaluating the effects of the novel GLP-1 analogue liraglutide in Alzheimer's disease: study protocol for a randomised controlled trial (ELAD study). Trials 2019;20(1):191.

142. Hou C, Lan J, Lin Y, et al. Chronic remote ischaemic conditioning in patients with symptomatic intracranial atherosclerotic stenosis (the RICA trial): a multicentre, randomised, double-blind sham-controlled trial in China. Lancet Neurol 2022; 21(12):1089–98.

143. Lahna D, Schwartz DL, Woltjer R, et al. Venous collagenosis as pathogenesis of white matter hyperintensity. Ann Neurol 2022;92(6):992–1000.

144. Houck AL, Gutierrez J, Gao F, et al. Increased diameters of the internal cerebral veins and the basal veins of rosenthal are associated with white matter hyperintensity volume. AJNR Am J Neuroradiol 2019;40(10):1712–8.

145. Moody DM, Brown WR, Challa VR, et al. Cerebral microvascular alterations in aging, leukoaraiosis, and Alzheimer's disease. Ann N Y Acad Sci 1997;826: 103–16.

146. Caplan LR. Lacunar infarction and small vessel disease: pathology and pathophysiology. J Stroke 2015;17(1):2–6.

147. Fang C, Magaki SD, Kim RC, et al. Arteriolar neuropathology in cerebral microvascular disease. Neuropathol Appl Neurobiol 2023;49(1):e12875.

148. Ungvari Z, Tarantini S, Kirkpatrick AC, et al. Cerebral microhemorrhages: mechanisms, consequences, and prevention. Am J Physiol Heart Circ Physiol 2017; 312(6):H1128–43.

149. Magaki S, Chen Z, Haeri M, et al. Charcot-Bouchard aneurysms revisited: clinicopathologic correlations. Mod Pathol 2021;34(12):2109–21.

150. Iliff J, Wang M, Liao Y, et al. A paravascular pathway facilitates CSF flow through the brain parenchyma and the clearance of interstitial solutes, including amyloid β. Sci Transl Med 2012;4(147).

151. Gouveia-Freitas K, Bastos-Leite AJ. Perivascular spaces and brain waste clearance systems: relevance for neurodegenerative and cerebrovascular pathology. Neuroradiology 2021;63(10):1581–97.

152. Bakker EN, Bacskai BJ, Arbel-Ornath M, et al. Lymphatic clearance of the brain: perivascular, paravascular and significance for neurodegenerative diseases. Cell Mol Neurobiol 2016;36(2):181–94.

153. Ramirez J, Berezuk C, McNeely AA, et al. Imaging the perivascular space as a potential biomarker of neurovascular and neurodegenerative diseases. Cell Mol Neurobiol 2016;36(2):289–99.

154. Martinez-Ramirez S, Pontes-Neto OM, Dumas AP, et al. Topography of dilated perivascular spaces in subjects from a memory clinic cohort. Neurology 2013; 80(17):1551–6.

155. Charidimou A, Meegahage R, Fox Z, et al. Enlarged perivascular spaces as a marker of underlying arteriopathy in intracerebral haemorrhage: a multicentre MRI cohort study. J Neurol Neurosurg Psychiatry 2013;84(6):624–9.

156. Charidimou A, Jaunmuktane Z, Baron J, et al. White matter perivascular spaces: an MRI marker in pathology-proven cerebral amyloid angiopathy? Neurology 2014;82(1):57–62.

157. De Kort AM, Kuiperij HB, Marques TM, et al. Decreased cerebrospinal fluid Abeta 38, 40, 42, and 43 levels in sporadic and hereditary cerebral amyloid angiopathy. Ann Neurol 2023. https://doi.org/10.1002/ana.26610.

158. Kaushik K, van Etten ES, Siegerink B, et al. Iatrogenic cerebral amyloid angiopathy post neurosurgery: frequency, clinical profile, radiological features, and outcome. Stroke 2023;54(5):1214–23.

159. Beaudin AE, McCreary CR, Mazerolle EL, et al. Cerebrovascular reactivity across the entire brain in cerebral amyloid angiopathy. Neurology 2022; 98(17):e1716–28.

Advances and Future Trends in the Diagnosis and Management of Intracerebral Hemorrhage

Christine E. Yeager, MD[a],*, Rajeev K. Garg, MD, MS[b]

KEYWORDS

- Intracerebral hemorrhage • Hemorrhagic stroke • Intraparenchymal hemorrhage

KEY POINTS

- Spontaneous intracerebral hemorrhage remains one of the deadliest forms of stroke despite advances in stroke and neurocritical care.
- Identifying predictors of poor outcomes and addressing therapeutic targets are active areas of research.
- Neuroimaging may play an important role in prognosis.
- Blood pressure control and reversal of coagulopathy are key components of medical management.
- Minimally minimal invasive surgery may provide a novel approach to improving outcomes in this disease.

INTRODUCTION
Epidemiology

Spontaneous intracerebral hemorrhage (sICH) accounts for approximately 10% to 15% of all strokes in the United States and remains one of the deadliest.[1] Between 2004 and 2018, the prevalence of ICH increased by 11% in the United States.[2] Of particular concern is that despite advances in neurocritical care and stroke, mortality remains high with 40% of patients dead at 1 month, and 54% dead at 1 year.[3,4] Morbidity also remains high, with only 12% to 39% of patients regaining long-term function independence.[4] Globally, sICH accounts for an estimated 5% of deaths annually which is equivalent to nearly 3 million deaths per year.[5]

[a] Division of Critical Care Neurology, Rush University Medical Center, 1725 W Harrison Street, Suite 1106, Chicago, IL, USA; [b] Division of Critical Care Neurology, Section of Cognitive Neurosciences, Rush University Medical Center, 1725 W Harrison Street, Suite 1106, Chicago, IL, USA
* Corresponding author.
E-mail address: Christine_e_yeager@rush.edu

Neurol Clin 42 (2024) 689–703
https://doi.org/10.1016/j.ncl.2024.03.004
neurologic.theclinics.com

Risk Factors

There are 2 main categories of sICH, primary versus secondary. Primary sICH accounts for over 85% of cases and is related to hypertension or cerebral amyloid angiopathy (CAA). The majority of primary sICH cases are attributed to hypertension.[6] Hypertensive arteriopathy predominantly affects small perforating arteries of the deep gray and deep white matter, while CAA results from the deposition of beta-amyloid within cortical and leptomeningeal arteries.[7] There is a new categorization called mixed ICH (both hypertensive and amyloid).[8] Secondary sICH can be related to multiple etiologies including coagulopathy, vascular abnormalities, substance use, neoplasms, or hemorrhagic conversion of ischemic infarcts. For all cases of sICH, studies have identified hypertension and anticoagulation use as the main risk factors.[9]

The increasing prevalence of sICH noted in the United States may be related to a greater prevalence of associated vascular risk factors. This observation may be driving the increased prevalence of sICH in younger demographics, which is concerning as this may extrapolate to higher health care care costs and loss of economic productivity.[2] Among patients hospitalized with intracerebral hemorrhage (ICH) there appears to be a higher prevalence of hypertension and anticoagulant use.[2] The highest incidence of ICH has been noted in non-Hispanic blacks; and it has been found that at the age of 45, non-Hispanic blacks had 5.8 times greater risk of sICH when compared to Caucasian patients of the same age.[2,10]

Outcomes

Identifying predictors of poor outcomes has been a long-standing area for research. The ICH score was developed and published in 2001 and its purpose was to provide providers with a framework for risk stratification and expected mortality; however, it was never meant to be used as a prognostic tool.[11] Additionally the ICH score was shown to overestimate mortality in patients that had full resuscitative efforts continued.[12] This has led studies to develop other prognostic scales and look at other clinical data for prognostication. The Functional Outcome in Patients with Primary Intracerebral Hemorrhage (FUNC) score was developed to control for the effect of the withdrawal of life-sustaining measures, as it was only applied to survivors of the sICH patients in their cohort and was found to be predictive of functional outcomes at 90 days.[13] However, further review of the FUNC score showed significant heterogeneity in outcomes at different time points, raising the concern that the initial findings may be related to chance rather than true predictive ability.[14]

Some studies noted that the location of the hemorrhage had significantly different outcomes, in terms of functional status and mortality with the thalamic and brainstem hemorrhages having worse outcomes when compared to lobar or other deep structures.[15] Multiple trials have identified hematoma expansion (HE) as a predictor of poor outcome; however, multiple clinical trials aimed at reducing HE have not reliably shown benefit.[16] Cognitive outcomes after sICH are still poorly defined. There have been studies evaluating the risk of dementia after ICH. One study found that early dementia is associated with hematoma size and location, with larger size and lobar location contributing greater risk.[17] The lobar location for ICH was also identified in another trial as a risk factor for developing dementia, suggesting that underlying CAA is a contributing factor to the development of new cognitive impairment.[18]

Ultimately more data are needed to address the therapeutic targets that have already been identified and more research is needed to identify additional prognostic factors, specifically factors that can be modified and treated, as this remains a challenge in this patient population and their identification could lead to improved patient outcomes.

Imaging

Early neuroimaging is necessary for the diagnosis of ICH. While computed tomography (CT) is still the most widely used modality due to availability and speed, MRI with gradient echo or susceptibility-weighted sequences has been shown to be very accurate in diagnosing hyperacute ICH.[19] There is growing literature on neuroimaging features that help predict patients who will have HE and worse functional outcomes in the long term.

Computed tomography

Irregular shape and heterogeneous density of hematomas on non-contrast CT scans have been predictive of hematoma growth.[20–22] Shape-related markers include the island sign and the satellite sign. The island sign (**Fig. 1**) is one of the more studied shape-related markers and it has been shown to be an independent predictor of HE, however, with lower accuracy than the CT angiography (CTA) spot sign.[23,24] Another shape-related imaging marker that has been suggested is the satellite sign (**Fig. 2**), but the relationship between this sign and HE remains not well defined.[25,26] Density-related markers include the blend sign, swirl sign, black hole sign, hypodensities, and fluid blood level. The blend sign (see **Fig. 1**) has a relatively low sensitivity (39.3%) for detecting HE; however, it was shown to have high specificity (95.5%).[27] Studies that have evaluated the swirl sign (**Fig. 3**) have found its presence potentially

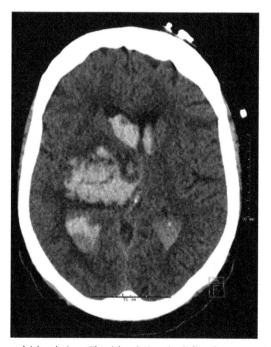

Fig. 1. Blend sign and island sign. The island sign is defined as an extremely irregularly shaped hematoma as seen in this figure.[23,24] The blend sign (*circle*) is identified by a low-density region with an adjacent high-density region within the hematoma separated by a well-defined margin, the difference in density between the 2 regions should be at least 18 Hounsfield units (Hu), and the low-density region should not be completely surrounded by the high-density region.[22]

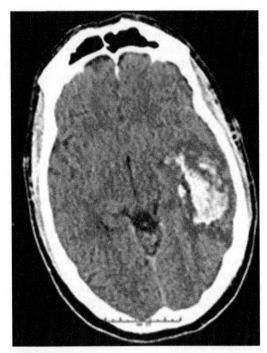

Fig. 2. Satellite sign, defined as high-density starry dots around the spontaneous intracerebral hemorrhage.[25,26]

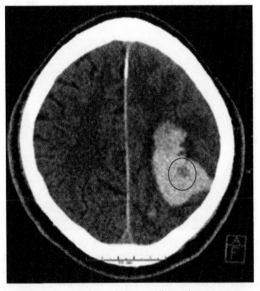

Fig. 3. Swirl sign, a hypodense or isodense lesion within a hyper-attenuated hematoma that can vary in shape.[22,28]

predicts poor functional outcomes and mortality; however, further studies are needed to assess its utility.[28] While some studies have suggested that the black hole sign (**Fig. 4**) may be predictive of worse clinical outcomes and association with HE, it was shown to be less accurate than the blend sign.[29]

According to American Heart Association (AHA) guidelines, CTA is recommended in patients with lobar sICH and age less than 70 years, deep/posterior fossa sICH and age less than 45 years, or deep/posterior fossa sICH in ages 45 to 70 years without a history of hypertension.[30] CTA can be useful for the prediction of HE and mortality as well.[31] In the PREDICT (Prediction of Haematoma Growth and Outcome in Patients with Intracerebral Haemorrhage Using the CT-Angiography Spot Sign) trial, patients with the CTA "spot sign" had significantly higher mortality at 3 months (43.4%) as compared to patients who were "spot sign" negative (19.6%)[32] (**Fig. 5**). CTA can also be used as part of the DIAGRAM (DIagnostic AngioGRAphy to find vascular Malformations) score to identify patients who are more likely to have a macrovascular cause of their ICH and may need further evaluation with digital subtraction angiography.[33]

MRI

MRI can help differentiate between primary and secondary sICH. Evidence of cerebral microbleeds may be indicative of CAA-related sICH, while chronic microvascular changes can be suggestive of underlying hypertension. Other etiologies such as cavernous malformation and malignancy can also be evident. In 2022, the Boston criteria 2.0 were published to incorporate emerging MRI markers on CAA.[34] The main MRI findings that led to this update were severe, MRI-visible centrum semiovale perivascular spaces and white matter hyperintensity patterns that seem to correlate with sICH etiology.[34] Studies have shown that severe perivascular spaces are more common in patients with proven CAA than non-CAA patients.[35]

There is also interest in leukoaraiosis patterns and the association with sICH, as it is more commonly present in patients with both ischemic strokes and sICH than in

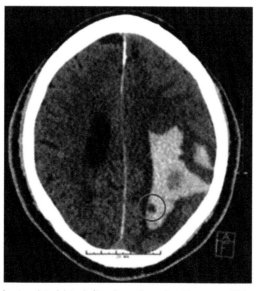

Fig. 4. The black hole sign (*circle*) is defined as a low-density area within a hematoma that is completely surrounded by the high-density hematoma.[22]

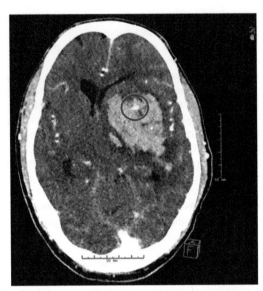

Fig. 5. Computed tomography angiography "spot sign." Note the focal extravasation of contrast containing blood within the hematoma.

healthy individuals. Leukoaraiosis is a feature of both hypertensive and CAA-related sICH.[36] In all stroke patients (ischemic and hemorrhagic), the presence of severe leukoaraiosis was associated with a higher risk of stroke (especially ischemic), higher mortality, and a higher risk of subsequent dementia.[37] There have been several studies that have noted that leukoaraiosis was associated with both worse functional outcomes and higher mortality in sICH patients.[38]

Another MRI feature that may be helpful in prognostication is the presence of diffusion-weighted imaging (DWI) lesions. DWI lesions remote from the hematoma itself can be found in 11% to 49% of patients with sICH and have been shown to be associated with increased morbidity and mortality.[39] DWI lesions have also been associated with increased risk for ischemic stroke and all-cause vascular events.[39,40] Data on the timing of these lesions suggest they occur 2 to 4 days after admission allowing them to be early radiographic prognostic biomarkers.[41] While the pathophysiology of these lesions remains unclear, growing evidence argues against failure of cerebral autoregulation during acute blood pressure reduction.[41]

Medical Management

Approximately one-third of patients with ICH experience HE within the first 3 hours.[42] Prevention of HE is one of the main targets of treatment, whether it be from blood pressure management, reversal of coagulopathy, or surgical intervention.[43] There is increasing interest in the use of bundled protocol that has been shown to be beneficial in a recent clinical trial.[44]

Blood pressure management

Optimal blood pressure targets in sICH continue to be somewhat debated. INTERACT2 (The Second Intensive Blood Pressure Reduction in Acute Cerebral Haemorrhage Trial) and ATACH-II (Antihypertensive Treatment of Acute Cerebral Hemorrhage-II) trials showed that intensive lowering of systolic blood pressure

(SBP) to less than 140 mm Hg when compared to lowering SBP to less than 180 mm Hg did not influence sICH outcomes.[45,46] ATACH-II showed that treatment of SBP in ICH to achieve110 to 130 mm Hg did not result in lower death or disability compared to those with the standard reduction to 140 to 179 mm Hg.[46] There was some suggestion of improvement in the SBP less than 140 mm Hg group; however, it was not significant. Another caveat was that in the ATACH-II trial, if presenting blood pressure was greater than 220 mm Hg, there was higher occurrence of neurologic dysfunction and adverse renal events in the intensive blood pressure–lowering group when blood pressure was reduced to less than 140 mm Hg.[46] Despite some differences in the trials, both showed rapid lowering of blood pressure to less than 140 mm Hg did not confer a mortality or morbidity benefit.[45,46] In addition, blood pressure lowering was not shown to prevent HE.[45,46] There are other data that SBP in general can be an unreliable target and there are many variables that affect its accuracy.[47] Accuracy of SBP in the intensive care unit is poor, and in ICH, SBP has been shown to be unreliable for managing and can vary based on the site of measurement and measurement dampening.[47–49] Mean arterial blood pressure (MAP) is thought to be a better marker of tissue perfusion so it may be a better target to analyze in future studies.[47] Overall, more evidence is needed to better delineate the ideal blood pressure targets, whether it be SBP, diastolic blood pressure, or MAP, and what the best agent is to achieve such targets.

Reversal of coagulopathy

Vitamin K antagonist reversal. Oral anticoagulation in ICH patients is associated with HE and higher mortality.[50] To mitigate HE, the priority of treatment is the emergent reversal of the coagulopathy. The management of warfarin reversal often includes a combination of vitamin K, fresh frozen plasma (FFP), and/or prothrombin complex concentrate (PCC) based on availability and protocols at each place of management. However, in a direct comparison, PCC is superior in terms of faster correction of the international normalized ratio, reduced HE, and improved mortality.[51,52] Additionally, in patients with concerns for volume overload, PCC may be preferred over FFP due to its smaller volume of administration.

Factor Xa inhibitor reversal. Direct factor Xa inhibitors are being used more commonly and the most feared complication is ICH. Andexanet alfa was developed as a specific reversal agent to mitigate the effects of both direct and indirect factor Xa inhibitors. The molecule is an inactive recombinant factor Xa modified to bind and inhibit direct and indirect FXa inhibition.[53,54] While andexanet alfa has been shown to provide good to excellent hemostatic efficacy and reverse the anti-Xa effect, there have been multiple smaller studies that have shown similar hemostatic efficacy and clinical outcomes with Andexanet alfa when compared to 4-factor PCC.[55–58] ANNEXA-1 (Trial of Andexanet in Patients Receiving an Oral FXa Inhibitor Who Require Urgent Surgery) was started to assess the efficacy and safety of andexanet alfa in patients on apixaban and rivaroxaban with intracranial hemorrhage. This trial was stopped early due to achieving the trial's criteria for superior hemostatic efficacy.[59] The authors are awaiting the results of the publication to further assess the impact on morbidity and mortality. Ciraparantag is a molecule that was designed to bind specifically to unfractionated heparin and low-molecular-weight heparins but there are also data to support that it can bind to and prevent the direct oral anticoagulants from binding with factor Xa.[60] It is currently still under investigation for its use in a clinical setting.

Direct thrombin inhibitors. Dabigatran is a selective, competitive, reversible direct thrombin inhibitor. Specific reversal of dabigatran is performed with idarucizumab, which is a monoclonal antibody that binds to dabigatran in an almost irreversible manner.[61] The RE-VERSE AD (A Study of the RE-VERSal Effects of Idarucizumab on Active Dabigatran) study evaluated the efficacy of idarucizumab in reversing dabigatran, and in the 503 patients they analyzed, anticoagulation was reversed rapidly and completely in over 98% of the patients; however, only 53 patients in this trial had sICH.[62] The effect of idarucizumab on HE is unknown at this time and further studies would be required to evaluate this further.

Antiplatelet reversal

Approximately a quarter of the patients with ICH are on antiplatelet therapy before their bleed occurrence.[63] There is controversy if the antiplatelet effect has been associated with early HE. Furthermore, in some studies, pre-ICH antiplatelet use was associated with worse outcomes, neurologic deterioration, death within 7 days, and death at 90 days.[63,64] Subgroup analysis of the TICH-2 (Tranexamic Acid to Improve Functional Status in Adults with Spontaneous Intracerebral Haemorrhage) trial data showed that pre-ICH antiplatelet use was associated with an increased risk of HE, neurologic decline, death, and poor functional outcomes.[64]

Desmopressin has been evaluated as well for use in antiplatelet-associated ICH; however, the data surrounding its use are conflicting. While some studies have shown improved platelet function after desmopressin administration in the setting of antiplatelet-related hemorrhages and decreased likelihood of HE,[45] others have shown no benefit in terms of preventing HE.[65–67] While the 2022 AHA guidelines make no recommendation regarding desmopressin due to uncertain efficacy, the guidelines from the Neurocritical Care Society from 2016 suggest consideration of a single dose of desmopressin due to low financial cost, low risk of harm, and small chance of potential benefit.[68]

Hemostatic therapies

There have been many studies looking at hemostatic therapies but as of now, there are no validated therapies. TICH-2 evaluated tranexamic acid (TXA) use in sICH, and while there was modest improvement in HE, there was overall no difference in functional outcomes at 90 days when compared to placebo.[69] However, this trial did show that TXA had a favorable safety profile and prompted additional studies using it within a shorter time frame from ICH onset.[69]

Recombinant factor VIIa has also been studied as a hemostatic therapy. The Recombinant Activated Factor VII for Acute Intracerebral Hemorrhage trial showed reduced hematoma growth and improved morbidity and mortality when recombinant factor VIIa was given within 4 hours of onset of sICH but did show an increase in thromboembolic adverse events.[70] This led to additional investigation; however, the FAST (Recombinant Factor VIIa in Acute Intracerebral Haemorrhage) trial, which was designed to test these results, did show reduced HE but did improve survival or functional outcome, and again showed an increase in arterial thromboembolic events.[71] Further evaluation of rFVIIa is ongoing with the National Institute of Neurological Disorders and Stroke–funded FASTEST trial (Recombinant Factor VIIa (rFVIIa) for Hemorrhagic Stroke Trial).

Bundled protocol approach

A single-center UK trial evaluated a bundle approach to the care of sICH patients incorporating blood pressure control, protocolized coagulopathy reversal, and a care pathway for neurosurgical intervention, and they noted lower 30-day mortality in ICH patients.[72] This trial was limited due to it not being randomized and the outcome was assessed after a short period rather than an extended assessment. INTERACT-3

(The Third, Intensive Care Bundle with Blood Pressure Reduction in Acute Cerebral Hemorrhage Trial) assessed a bundle approach for patients with ICH incorporating algorithms for hyperglycemia, fever control, and abnormal coagulation, and this bundled approach resulted in improved functional outcomes at 6 months in low-income and middle-income countries.[44]

Anti-seizure medications

The incidence of seizures may still be unclear; however, some studies have shown it in at least one-third of patients who present with ICH.[73] Majority of the seizures that occur do so within the first 24 hours of the hemorrhage; however, despite the relatively high frequency of seizures in this patient population, the use of prophylactic anti-seizure medications is not supported by evidence at this time.[74,75] Decision-making becomes more complex as it is estimated that around 50% of seizures after sICH are only detectable electrographically.[73] Electroencephalogram can be considered in patients with unexplained abnormal mental status and should be considered for a duration longer than 24 hours.[73]

Surgical Management

Surgical evacuation of hematomas has been evaluated with several studies and while there are often suggestions of treatment effects, it has not been shown to improve patient outcomes. There is increasing interest in using minimally invasive surgery (MIS) early in ICH to reduce the mass effect and prevent the secondary neuronal injury that may occur with breakdown of blood products. Craniotomy or craniectomy have been evaluated in the past with several trials; the main randomized control trials that are referenced are STICH (Early Surgery versus Initial Conservative Treatment in Patients with Spontaneous Supratentorial Intracerebral Haematomas in the International Surgical Trial in Intracerebral Haemorrhage) and STICH-II (Early surgery versus initial conservative treatment in patients with spontaneous supratentorial lobar intracerebral haematomas), which failed to show benefit of surgery over medical management alone but had some suggestions that surgery could benefit the subgroup of patients with a superficial ICH.[76,77] MIS has had more interest due to the goal of reducing damage to healthy brain tissue. Many prior trials had not shown mortality benefit for surgery when compared with conventional medical therapy; however, MISTIE III (Minimally Invasive Surgery plus Rt-PA for ICH Evacuation Phase III) did show lower mortality with MIS when compared with medical therapy.[78] However, the primary endpoint of MISTIE-III was evaluating functional outcomes in using the MISTIE protocol versus medical management, and this was not shown to be significantly different.[78]

Clot removal with thrombolysis in intraventricular hemorrhage has also been evaluated due to its association with higher morbidity and mortality. Thrombolysis of clot burden with intravenous tissue-type plasminogen activator (IV tPA) was shown to be safe via an external ventricular drain so it was hypothesized that it would improve functional outcomes in patients.[78] CLEAR III (Clot Lysis: Evaluating Accelerated Resolution of Intraventricular Hemorrhage Phase III) evaluated this hypothesis and was unable to show improvement in functional outcomes with the administration of IV tPA via an external ventricular drain.[79] Further studies will need to be considered, however, as there was a suggestion of value in removing larger amounts of clot burden.[79]

Recently released positive results from the ENRICH (Early MiNimally-invasive Removal of IntraCerebral Hemorrhage) trial may change the surgical approach in sICH; however, the data from the trial will need to be reviewed when it becomes available. Another minimally invasive trial, the MIND (Artemis in the Removal of

Intracerebral Hemorrhage) trial utilizing the Artemis neuro evacuation device is currently ongoing as well, with expected completion in 2028.

Future Investigation

- Developing imaging markers for predicting worse outcomes and HE
- Developing scores to predict outcome
- Hemostatic therapies
- MIS

CLINICS CARE POINTS

- ICH incidence is increasing due to increasing prevalence of uncontrolled hypertension in the younger patient population.
- MRI findings may help provide prognostic data and help guide clinical decisions.
- Blood pressure management is still one of the mainstays of medical management; however, the ideal target is still being evaluated and further studies should be performed to assess MAP over SBP.
- MIS remains of significant interest especially with the first positive trial soon to be published.

DISCLOSURE

The authors have no disclosures.

REFERENCES

1. Tsao CW, Aday AW, Almarzooq ZI, et al. Heart disease and stroke Statistics—2022 update: A report from the american heart association. Circulation 2022; 145(8):e153–639. Available at: https://www.ncbi.nlm.nih.gov/pubmed/35078371.
2. Bako AT, Pan A, Potter T, et al. Contemporary trends in the nationwide incidence of primary intracerebral hemorrhage. Stroke 2022;53(3):e70–4. Available at: https://www.ncbi.nlm.nih.gov/pubmed/35109682.
3. Pinho J, Costa AS, Araújo JM, et al. Intracerebral hemorrhage outcome: A comprehensive update. J Neurol Sci 2019;398:54–66.
4. van Asch CJ,MD, Luitse MJ,MD, Rinkel GJ,MD, et al. MD. Incidence, case fatality, and functional outcome of intracerebral haemorrhage over time, according to age, sex, and ethnic origin: A systematic review and meta-analysis. Lancet Neurol 2010;9(2):167–76. Available at: https://www.clinicalkey.es/playcontent/1-s2.0-S1474442209703400.
5. GBD 2017 Disease and Injury Incidence and Prevalence Collaborators. Global, regional, and national incidence, prevalence, and years lived with disability for 354 diseases and injuries for 195 countries and territories, 1990-2017: A systematic analysis for the global burden of disease study 2017. 2018. Available at: https://www.repository.cam.ac.uk/handle/1810/296929.
6. Flower O, Smith M. The acute management of intracerebral hemorrhage. Curr Opin Crit Care 2011;17(2):106–14. Available at: https://www.ncbi.nlm.nih.gov/pubmed/21169826.
7. Charidimou A, Boulouis G, Haley K, et al. White matter hyperintensity patterns in cerebral amyloid angiopathy and hypertensive arteriopathy. Neurology 2016; 86(6):505–11. Available at: https://www.ncbi.nlm.nih.gov/pubmed/26747886.

8. Pasi M, Charidimou A, Boulouis G, et al. Mixed-location cerebral hemorrhage/microbleeds: Underlying microangiopathy and recurrence risk. Neurology 2018; 90(2):e119–26. Available at: https://www.ncbi.nlm.nih.gov/pubmed/29247070.

9. Martini SR, Flaherty ML, Broderick JP, et al. Risk factors for intracerebral hemorrhage differ according to hemorrhage location. Neurology 2012;79(23):2275–82. Available at: https://www.ncbi.nlm.nih.gov/pubmed/23175721.

10. HOWARD G, CUSHMAN M, HOWARD VJ, et al. Risk factors for intracerebral hemorrhage the REasons for geographic and racial differences in stroke (REGARDS) study. Stroke 2013;44(5):1282–7. Available at: https://www.ncbi.nlm.nih.gov/pubmed/23532012.

11. Hemphill 3 JC, Bonovich DC, Besmertis L, et al. The ICH score: A simple, reliable grading scale for intracerebral hemorrhage. Stroke 2001;32(4):891–7. Available at: https://www.ncbi.nlm.nih.gov/pubmed/11283388.

12. Zahuranec DB, Brown DL, Lisabeth LD, et al. Early care limitations independently predict mortality after intracerebral hemorrhage. Neurology 2007;68(20):1651–7. Available at: https://www.ncbi.nlm.nih.gov/pubmed/17502545.

13. Rost NS, Smith EE, Chang Y, et al. Prediction of functional outcome in patients with primary intracerebral hemorrhage: The FUNC score. Stroke 2008;39(8): 2304–9. Available at: http://stroke.ahajournals.org/cgi/content/abstract/39/8/2304.

14. Gregório T, Pipa S, Cavaleiro P, et al. Assessment and comparison of the four most extensively validated prognostic scales for intracerebral hemorrhage: Systematic review with meta-analysis. Neurocritical Care 2019;30(2):449–66. Available at: https://link.springer.com/article/10.1007/s12028-018-0633-6.

15. Teo K, Fong S, Leung WCY, et al. Location-specific hematoma volume cutoff and clinical outcomes in intracerebral hemorrhage. Stroke (1970) 2023;54(6): 1548–57. Available at: https://www.ncbi.nlm.nih.gov/pubmed/37216445.

16. Morotti A, Boulouis G, Dowlatshahi D, et al. Intracerebral haemorrhage expansion: Definitions, predictors, and prevention. Lancet Neurol 2023;22(2):159–71.

17. Biffi A, Bailey D, Anderson CD, et al. Risk factors associated with early vs delayed dementia after intracerebral hemorrhage. JAMA Neurol 2016;73(8):969–76.

18. Moulin S,MD, Labreuche J, Bst Bombois S, PhD, Boulouis G, Hénon H, Duhamel A, Leys D, Cordonnier C. Dementia risk after spontaneous intracerebral haemorrhage: A prospective cohort study. Lancet Neurol 2016;15(8):820–9. Available at: https://www.clinicalkey.es/playcontent/1-s2.0-S1474442216001307.

19. Fiebach JB, Schellinger PD, Gass A, et al. Stroke magnetic resonance imaging is accurate in hyperacute intracerebral hemorrhage: A multicenter study on the validity of stroke imaging. Stroke 2004;35(2):502–6. Available at: http://stroke.ahajournals.org/cgi/content/abstract/35/2/502.

20. Barras CD, Tress BM, Christensen S, et al. Density and shape as CT predictors of intracerebral hemorrhage growth. Stroke 2009;40(4):1325–31. Available at: http://stroke.ahajournals.org/cgi/content/abstract/40/4/1325.

21. Morotti A, Boulouis G, Dowlatshahi D, et al. Standards for detecting, interpreting, and reporting noncontrast computed tomographic markers of intracerebral hemorrhage expansion. Ann Neurol 2019;86(4):480–92. Available at: https://onlinelibrary.wiley.com/doi/abs/10.1002/ana.25563.

22. Huang Y, Huang H, Li Z, et al. Research advances in imaging markers for predicting hematoma expansion in intracerebral hemorrhage: A narrative review. Front Neurol 2023;14:1176390. Available at: https://www.ncbi.nlm.nih.gov/pubmed/37181553.

23. Li Q, Liu Q, Yang W, et al. Island sign: An imaging predictor for early hematoma expansion and poor outcome in patients with intracerebral hemorrhage. Stroke 2017;48(11):3019–25. Available at: https://www.ncbi.nlm.nih.gov/pubmed/29018128.

24. Zheng J, Yu Z, Wang C, et al. Evaluating the predictive value of island sign and spot sign for hematoma expansion in spontaneous intracerebral hemorrhage. World neurosurgery 2018;117:e167–71.

25. Huang Y, Huang H, Li Z, et al. Research advances in imaging markers for predicting hematoma expansion in intracerebral hemorrhage: A narrative review. Front Neurol 2023;14:1176390. https://doi.org/10.3389/fneur.2023.1176390. Available at: https://www.ncbi.nlm.nih.gov/pubmed/37181553.

26. Shimoda Y, Ohtomo S, Arai H, et al. Satellite sign: A poor outcome predictor in intracerebral hemorrhage. Cerebrovascular diseases (Basel, Switzerland) 2017; 44(3–4):105–12. Available at: https://www.ncbi.nlm.nih.gov/pubmed/28605739.

27. Li Q, Zhang G, Huang Y, et al. Blend sign on computed tomography: Novel and reliable predictor for early hematoma growth in patients with intracerebral hemorrhage. Stroke 2015;46(8):2119–23. Available at: https://www.ncbi.nlm.nih.gov/pubmed/26089330.

28. Amoo M, Henry J, Alabi PO, et al. The 'swirl sign' as a marker for haematoma expansion and outcome in intra-cranial haemorrhage: A meta-analysis. J Clin Neurosci 2021;87:103–11.

29. Li R, Yang M. A comparative study of the blend sign and the black hole sign on CT as a predictor of hematoma expansion in spontaneous intracerebral hemorrhage. BioScience Trends 2017;11(6):682–7. Available at: https://www.jstage.jst.go.jp/article/bst/11/6/11_2017.01283/_article/-char/en.

30. Greenberg SM, Ziai WC, Cordonnier C, et al. 2022 guideline for the management of patients with spontaneous intracerebral hemorrhage: A guideline from the american heart association/american stroke association. Stroke 2022;53(7): e361. Available at: https://www.ncbi.nlm.nih.gov/pubmed/35579034.

31. Rizos T, Dörner N, Jenetzky E, et al. Spot signs in intracerebral hemorrhage: Useful for identifying patients at risk for hematoma enlargement? Cerebrovascular diseases (Basel, Switzerland) 2013;35(6):582–9. Available at: https://www.karger.com/Article/Abstract/348851.

32. Demchuk Andrew M, Dr Prof, Dowlatshahi D, Blas YS, Dzialowski I, Kobayashi A, Boulanger JM, Lum C, Gubitz G, Padma V, Roy J, Kase CS, Kosior J, Bhatia R, Tymchuk S, Subramaniam S, Gladstone DJ, Hill MD, Aviv RI, PREDICT/Sunnybrook ICH CTA study groupMD, Rodriguez-Luna D. Prediction of haematoma growth and outcome in patients with intracerebral haemorrhage using the CT-angiography spot sign (PREDICT): A prospective observational study. Lancet Neurol 2012;11(4):307–14. Available at: https://www.clinicalkey.es/playcontent/1-s2.0-S1474442212700388.

33. Hilkens NA, van Asch CJJ, Werring DJ, et al. Predicting the presence of macrovascular causes in non-traumatic intracerebral haemorrhage: The DIAGRAM prediction score. J Neurol Neurosurg Psychiatry 2018;89(7):674–9.

34. Charidimou A, Boulouis G, Frosch MP, et al. The boston criteria version 2.0 for cerebral amyloid angiopathy: A multicentre, retrospective, MRI–neuropathology diagnostic accuracy study. Lancet Neurol 2022;21(8):714–25.

35. Charidimou A, Jaunmuktane Z, Baron J, et al. White matter perivascular spaces: An MRI marker in pathology-proven cerebral amyloid angiopathy? Neurology 2014;82(1):57–62. Available at: https://www.ncbi.nlm.nih.gov/pubmed/24285616.

36. Smith EE. Leukoaraiosis and stroke. Stroke (1970) 2010;41(10 Suppl):S139–43. Available at: https://www.ncbi.nlm.nih.gov/pubmed/20876490.
37. DEBETTE S, BEISER A, DECARLI C, et al. Association of MRI markers of vascular brain injury with incident stroke, mild cognitive impairment, dementia and mortality: The framingham offspring study. Stroke 2010;41(4):600–6. Available at: https://www.ncbi.nlm.nih.gov/pubmed/20167919.
38. Yu Z, Zheng J, Guo R, et al. Prognostic significance of leukoaraiosis in intracerebral hemorrhage: A meta-analysis. J Neurol Sci 2019;397:34–41.
39. Boulanger M, Schneckenburger R, Join-Lambert C, et al. Diffusion-weighted imaging hyperintensities in subtypes of acute intracerebral hemorrhage: Meta-analysis. Stroke 2019;50(1):135–42.
40. Garg RK, Khan J, Dawe RJ, et al. The influence of diffusion weighted imaging lesions on outcomes in patients with acute spontaneous intracerebral hemorrhage. Neurocritical Care 2020;33(2):552–64. Available at: https://link.springer.com/article/10.1007/s12028-020-00933-3.
41. Garg RK, Alberawi M, Ouyang B, et al. Timing of diffusion weighted imaging lesions in spontaneous intracerebral hemorrhage. J Neurol Sci 2021;425:117434.
42. Al-Shahi Salman R, Frantzias J, Lee RJ, et al. Absolute risk and predictors of the growth of acute spontaneous intracerebral haemorrhage: A systematic review and meta-analysis of individual patient data. Lancet Neurol 2018;17(10):885–94.
43. Selim M, Hanley D, Steiner T, et al. Recommendations for clinical trials in ICH: The second hemorrhagic stroke academia industry roundtable. Stroke 2020;51(4):1333–8. Available at: https://www.narcis.nl/publication/RecordID/oai:repository.ubn.ru.nl:2066%2F220280.
44. Ma L, Ouyang M, Malavera A, et al. The third intensive care bundle with blood pressure reduction in acute cerebral haemorrhage trial (INTERACT3): An international, stepped wedge cluster randomised controlled trial. The Lancet (British edition) 2023;402(10395):27–40.
45. Anderson CS, Heeley E, Huang Y, et al. Rapid blood-pressure lowering in patients with acute intracerebral hemorrhage. N Engl J Med 2013;368(25):2355–65. Available at: https://nejm.org/doi/full/10.1056/NEJMoa1214609.
46. Qureshi AI, Palesch YY, Barsan WG, et al. Intensive blood-pressure lowering in patients with acute cerebral hemorrhage. N Engl J Med 2016;375(11):1033–43. Available at: https://nejm.org/doi/full/10.1056/NEJMoa1603460.
47. Garg RK, Ouyang B, Zwein A, et al. Systolic blood pressure measurements are unreliable for the management of acute spontaneous intracerebral hemorrhage. J Crit Care 2022;70:154049.
48. RAMSEY MI. Blood pressure monitoring: Automated oscil-lometric devices. J Clin Monit 1991;7(1):56–67. Available at: https://www.ncbi.nlm.nih.gov/pubmed/1999699.
49. Henry JB, Miller MC, Kelly KC, et al. Mean arterial pressure (MAP): An alternative and preferable measurement to systolic blood pressure (SBP) in patients for hypotension detection during hemapheresis. J Clin Apher 2002;17(2):55–64. Available at: https://api.istex.fr/ark:/67375/WNG-JG55XJS9-7/fulltext.pdf.
50. Cucchiara B, Messe S, Sansing L, et al. Hematoma growth in oral anticoagulant related intracerebral hemorrhage. Stroke 2008;39(11):2993–6. Available at: http://stroke.ahajournals.org/cgi/content/abstract/39/11/2993.
51. Hill R, Han TS, Lubomirova I, et al. Prothrombin complex concentrates are superior to fresh frozen plasma for emergency reversal of vitamin K antagonists: A meta-analysis in 2606 subjects. Drugs 2019;79(14):1557–65. Available at: https://link.springer.com/article/10.1007/s40265-019-01179-w.

52. Steiner T, Poli S, Griebe M, et al. Fresh frozen plasma versus prothrombin complex concentrate in patients with intracranial haemorrhage related to vitamin K antagonists (INCH): A randomised trial. Lancet Neurol 2016;15(6):566–73. Available at: https://www.clinicalkey.es/playcontent/1-s2.0-S1474442216001101.

53. Smythe M, Trujillo T, Fanikos J. Reversal agents for use with direct and indirect anticoagulants. Am J Health Syst Pharm 2016;73(10 Suppl 2):S27–48. Available at: http://ovidsp.ovid.com/ovidweb.cgi?T=JS&NEWS=n&CSC=Y&PAGE=full text&D=ovft&AN=00043627-201605152-00004.

54. Siegal DM, Curnutte JT, Connolly SJ, et al. Andexanet alfa for the reversal of factor xa inhibitor activity. N Engl J Med 2015;373(25):2413–24. Available at: https://nejm.org/doi/full/10.1056/NEJMoa1510991.

55. Connolly SJ, Crowther M, Eikelboom JW, et al. Full study report of andexanet alfa for bleeding associated with factor xa inhibitors. N Engl J Med 2019. https://doi.org/10.1056/NEJMoa1814051. Available at: http://hdl.handle.net/2078.1/225570.

56. Giovino A, Shomo E, Busey KV, et al. An 18-month single-center observational study of real-world use of andexanet alfa in patients with factor xa inhibitor associated intracranial hemorrhage. Clin Neurol Neurosurg 2020;195:106070.

57. Ammar AA, Ammar MA, Owusu KA, et al. Andexanet alfa versus 4-factor prothrombin complex concentrate for reversal of factor xa inhibitors in intracranial hemorrhage. Neurocritical Care 2021;35(1):255–61. Available at: https://link.springer.com/article/10.1007/s12028-020-01161-5.

58. Barra ME, Das AS, Hayes BD, et al. Evaluation of andexanet alfa and four-factor prothrombin complex concentrate (4F-PCC) for reversal of rivaroxaban- and apixaban-associated intracranial hemorrhages. J Thromb Haemostasis 2020;18(7): 1637–47. Available at: https://onlinelibrary.wiley.com/doi/abs/10.1111/jth.14838.

59. Trial of andexanet alfa in ICrH patients receiving an oral FXa inhibitor. ClinicalTrials.gov website Web site. 2023. Available at: https://clinicaltrials.gov/study/NCT03661528. [Accessed 12 July 2023].

60. Ansell J, Laulicht BE, Bakhru SH, et al. Ciraparantag, an anticoagulant reversal drug: Mechanism of action, pharmacokinetics, and reversal of anticoagulants. Blood 2021;137(1):115–25.

61. Kuramatsu JB, Sembill JA, Huttner HB. Reversal of oral anticoagulation in patients with acute intracerebral hemorrhage. Crit Care 2019;23(1):206. Available at: https://www.ncbi.nlm.nih.gov/pubmed/31171018.

62. Pollack CV, Reilly PA, van Ryn J, et al. Idarucizumab for dabigatran reversal — full cohort analysis. N Engl J Med 2017;377(5):431–41. Available at: https://nejm.org/doi/full/10.1056/NEJMoa1707278.

63. Thompson BB, Bejor Y, Hallevi H, et al. Prior antiplatelet therapy and outcome following intracerebral hemorrhage: A systematic review. Neurology 2010; 75(15):1333–42. Available at: https://www.ncbi.nlm.nih.gov/pubmed/20826714.

64. Law ZK, Desborough M, Roberts I, et al. Outcomes in Antiplatelet-Associated intracerebral hemorrhage in the TICH-2 randomized controlled trial. J Am Heart Assoc 2021;10(5):e019130. Available at: https://www.ncbi.nlm.nih.gov/pubmed/33586453.

65. Naidech AM, Maas MB, Levasseur-Franklin KE, et al. Desmopressin improves platelet activity in acute intracerebral hemorrhage. Stroke 2014;45(8):2451–3. Available at: https://www.ncbi.nlm.nih.gov/pubmed/25005444.

66. Mengel A, Stefanou M, Hadaschik K, et al. Early administration of desmopressin and platelet transfusion for reducing hematoma expansion in patients with acute antiplatelet therapy associated intracerebral hemorrhage. Crit Care Med 2020; 48(7):1009–17. Available at: https://www.ncbi.nlm.nih.gov/pubmed/32304415.

67. Schmidt KJ, Sager B, Zachariah J, et al. Cohort analysis of desmopressin effect on hematoma expansion in patients with spontaneous intracerebral hemorrhage and documented pre-ictus antiplatelet use. J Clin Neurosci 2019;66:33–7.

68. Frontera J, Lewin J, Rabinstein A, et al. Guideline for reversal of antithrombotics in intracranial hemorrhage: Executive summary. A statement for healthcare professionals from the neurocritical care society and the society of critical care medicine. Crit Care Med 2016;44(12):2251–7. Available at: http://ovidsp.ovid.com/ovidweb.cgi?T=JS&NEWS=n&CSC=Y&PAGE=fulltext&D=ovft&AN=00003246-201612000-00016.

69. Sprigg N, Flaherty K, Appleton JP, et al. Tranexamic acid for hyperacute primary IntraCerebral haemorrhage (TICH-2): An international randomised, placebo-controlled, phase 3 superiority trial. Lancet (London, England) 2018;391(10135):2107–15.

70. Mayer SA, Brun NC, Begtrup K, et al. Recombinant activated factor VII for acute intracerebral hemorrhage. N Engl J Med 2005;352(8):777–85. Available at: http://content.nejm.org/cgi/content/abstract/352/8/777.

71. Mayer SA, Brun NC, Begtrup K, et al. Efficacy and safety of recombinant activated factor VII for acute intracerebral hemorrhage. N Engl J Med 2008;358(20):2127–37. Available at: http://content.nejm.org/cgi/content/abstract/358/20/2127.

72. Parry-Jones AR, Sammut-Powell C, Paroutoglou K, et al. An intracerebral hemorrhage care bundle is associated with lower case fatality. Ann Neurol 2019;86(4):495–503. Available at: https://onlinelibrary.wiley.com/doi/abs/10.1002/ana.25546.

73. CLAASSEN J, JETTE N, MAYER SA, et al. Electrographic seizures and periodic discharges after intracerebral hemorrhage. Neurology 2007;69(13):1356–65. Available at: https://www.ncbi.nlm.nih.gov/pubmed/17893296.

74. Messé SR, Sansing LH, Cucchiara BL, et al, CHANT investigators. Prophylactic antiepileptic drug use is associated with poor outcome following ICH. Neurocritical Care 2009;11(1):38–44. Available at: https://link.springer.com/article/10.1007/s12028-009-9207-y.

75. Naidech AM, Garg RK, Liebling S, et al. Anticonvulsant use and outcomes after intracerebral hemorrhage. Stroke 2009;40(12):3810–5. Available at: http://stroke.ahajournals.org/cgi/content/abstract/40/12/3810.

76. Mendelow AD, Gregson BA, Fernandes HM, et al. Early surgery versus initial conservative treatment in patients with spontaneous supratentorial intracerebral haematomas in the international surgical trial in intracerebral haemorrhage (STICH): A randomised trial. Lancet (British edition) 2005;365(9457):387–97. Available at: https://www.ncbi.nlm.nih.gov/pubmed/15680453.

77. Mendelow AD, Gregson BA, Rowan EN, et al, STICH II Investigators. FRCS. Early surgery versus initial conservative treatment in patients with spontaneous supratentorial lobar intracerebral haematomas (STICH II): A randomised trial. Lancet 2013;382(9890):397–408. Available at: https://www.clinicalkey.es/playcontent/1-s2.0-S0140673613609861.

78. Thompson RE, Lane K, Mayo SW, et al. Efficacy and safety of minimally invasive surgery with thrombolysis in intracerebral haemorrhage evacuation (MISTIE III): A randomised, controlled, open-label, blinded endpoint phase 3 trial. The Lancet (British edition) 2019;393(10175):1021–32.

79. Hanley DF, Lane K, CMAMcBee N, et al. Thrombolytic removal of intraventricular haemorrhage in treatment of severe stroke: Results of the randomised, multicentre, multiregion, placebo-controlled CLEAR III trial. The Lancet (British edition) 2017;389(10069):603–11. Available at: https://www.clinicalkey.es/playcontent/1-s2.0-S0140673616324102.

Advances and Future Trends in the Diagnosis and Management of Subarachnoid Hemorrhage

Giuseppe Lanzino, MD[a,b,*], Alejandro A. Rabinstein, MD[c]

KEYWORDS

- Aneurysmal subarachnoid hemorrhage • Hydrocephalus • Intracranial pressure
- Rebleeding • Vasospasm

KEY POINTS

- Treatment of a patient with aneurysmal subarachnoid hemorrhage is based on lessening the effects of the primary bleed while preventing secondary damage from its neurologic and medical complications.
- Euvolemia, correction of hyponatremia and other medical complications, and close neurologic monitoring are critical during the period of high risk for vasospasm since patients are very sensitive to secondary damage during this interval.
- Tight control of intracranial pressure in aneurysmal subarachnoid hemorrhage to levels lower than those considered safe in traumatic brain injury is emerging as an important factor in minimizing the effects of vasospasm, thereby improving outcomes.
- The decision about the best therapeutic modality to obliterate a ruptured aneurysm in a given patient is nuanced and, ideally, should be determined by a multidisciplinary team with expertise in neurocritical care, endovascular techniques, and microneurosurgery.

INTRODUCTION

Despite improvements in neurocritical care, endovascular, and open neurosurgery, aneurysmal subarachnoid hemorrhage (aSAH) remains one of the most challenging diseases in acute vascular neurology.[1] Treatment of patient with aSAH is focused on lessening the primary effects of the original bleed and preventing a secondary injury from its medical and neurologic complications (eg, rebleeding, vasospasm, hydrocephalus,

[a] Department of Neurological Surgery, Mayo Clinic, 200 First Street Southwest, Rochester, MN 55905, USA; [b] Department of Radiology, Mayo Clinic, 200 First Street Southwest, Rochester, MN 55905, USA; [c] Department of Neurology, Mayo Clinic, 200 First Street SW, Rochester, MN 55905, USA
* Corresponding author. Department of Neurological Surgery, Mayo Clinic, 200 First Street Southwest, Rochester, MN 55905.
E-mail address: lanzino.giuseppe@mayo.edu

Neurol Clin 42 (2024) 705–716
https://doi.org/10.1016/j.ncl.2024.03.005
0733-8619/24/© 2024 Elsevier Inc. All rights reserved.

neurologic.theclinics.com

and increased intracranial pressure [ICP]). The recent history of the treatment of this disease has been characterized by excitement for newer and often quite aggressive and intensive medical interventions, only to realize that in most circumstances, "less is more." Comprehensive guidelines of the American Heart Association (AHA)[2] on the management of aSAH have been published this past year, but major knowledge gaps remain, as highlighted by the recent aSAH guidelines from the Neurocritical Care Society.[3] The present article focuses on several areas of controversy and potential future development.

INITIAL DIAGNOSIS AND MANAGEMENT

Head computerized tomography (CT) remains the main diagnostic study to confirm the diagnosis of SAH. With modern scanners, a head CT done within 6 hours of symptom onset and interpreted by a board-certified neuroradiologist is sufficient to confirm or exclude SAH.[2] In patients with a high index of suspicion, CT can be combined with CT angiography for characterization of the possible underlying vascular pathology. For patients with acute severe headache who present to medical attention more than 6 hours after symptom onset, a lumbar puncture to exclude xanthochromia remains the next test of choice. MRI is still impractical and of untested value in the acute diagnosis of SAH. In patients with multiple aneurysms, understanding which aneurysm bled can be challenging at times. Laterality of blood on head CT and morphologic features of the aneurysm (presence of secondary lobulations, irregularity, and size) are factors which aid in identifying the ruptured aneurysm. In such cases, aneurysm wall enhancement has also been shown to help identify the ruptured aneurysm,[4] though this promising technique remains in its infancy.

There is often a major focus on systemic blood pressure control in the acute phase after aSAH. One of the most consistent systemic consequences of aneurysm rupture is a sudden rise in blood pressure. This observation has led some to erroneously conclude that high blood pressure is associated with increased risk of aneurysm rerupture, even though there is no evidence to support this statement. As a result, the most recent guidelines are quite cautious about recommending specific blood pressure goals.[2,3] However, hypotension must be avoided in the setting of increased ICP, as it leads to parenchymal ischemia. Anecdotally, we have observed over the years a few patients in the hyperacute phase who have experienced rebleeding in the setting of Valsalva maneuvers (ie, holding their breath during catheter angiography to optimize picture quality in awake patients, reacting to pain and discomfort during Foley catheter insertion, etc.). Thus, our experience suggests that a Valsalva maneuver, rather than systemic hypertension, may be associated with rebleeding. The mechanism would be a transient slowing/arrest of flow during Valsalva because of the increase in resistance to venous outflow, leading to increased ICP, followed by the sudden release which may cause sudden hemodynamic changes in the freshly ruptured aneurysm.

Clinically diagnosing seizures at presentation after SAH can be difficult. In patients without clear-cut seizures, there is consensus that prophylactic anticonvulsants are not indicated.[2] However, several patients who lose consciousness at the time of the initial bleed may present with seizurelike generalized tonic–clonic movements. These are considered to be the expression of near-complete or complete transient cerebral blood flow arrest occurring shortly after aneurysm rupture when the sudden rise in ICP reaches a level equaling perfusion pressure. Seizures occurring after the immediate acute phase when a patient has been stabilized but the aneurysm has not yet been secured are often the expression of rebleeding or worsening hydrocephalus. Anticonvulsants should be administered for 7 days to patients who have suffered a documented seizure,[2] while prophylactic anticonvulsants (a common practice throughout most units not long ago) are not indicated. There is some evidence that phenytoin may worsen outcomes, and it is less tolerated than levetiracetam.[5,6]

PREVENTION OF REBLEEDING

Aneurysm rebleeding is a devastating event often associated with poor prognosis.[7] The best way to prevent acute rebleeding is by treating the offending aneurysm. The incidence of rebleeding is high in the first 6 to 12 hours after aSAH and much lower afterward. This has important practical implications: patients evaluated in the local emergency department are at much higher risk of rebleeding (and potentially benefit from ultra-early aneurysm treatment) than those transferred to a tertiary referral center after being stabilized in an outside facility. Thus, while a policy of ultra-early aneurysm treatment to prevent rebleeding may make sense for patients admitted through the local ED, it is not effective for those transferred from outside facilities. In a recent analysis of a contemporary cohort of 317 patients with SAH evaluated over a 4 year interval (2010–2014), 60.9% of the rebleeding episodes occurred prior to admission to the authors' tertiary referral center.[8] Thus, the authors concluded that in their facility, a policy of ultra-early aneurysm obliteration, defined as treatment within 24 hours, would have prevented only 1 in 24 (4.2%) of the rebleeding episodes observed. Of note, the term "ultra-early," often used in the literature to categorize aneurysm treatment within 24 hours of aSAH diagnosis, may lead to incorrect interpretations. Rushing patients to have the ruptured aneurysm secured is not safe until the patient has been stabilized. There is no evidence that aneurysm treatment within the first 6 to 12 hours improves clinical outcomes.[9]

Pharmacologic therapy, in particular the utilization of antifibrinolytic drugs, has been evaluated in depth. In the 1980s, when delayed surgery was the modus operandi, randomized studies had shown that antifibrinolytic therapy (usually administered through continuous intravenous [IV] infusion) was beneficial in reducing the incidence of rebleeding at the expense of higher rates of vasospasm and hydrocephalus, presumably because of the reduced clearance of blood from the subarachnoid space.[10] As early aneurysm treatment became the standard of care for most patients, antifibrinolytic drugs were no longer used. However, results of a relatively small Scandinavian study of IV boluses of tranexamic acid administered immediately after diagnosis and every 6 hours until aneurysm treatment (or for up to 72 hours) suggested a benefit on early rebleeding.[11] Their results led to a re-evaluation of such pharmacologic intervention, which was eventually widely adopted. A recent multicenter randomized clinical trial, however, has challenged this practice. In this trial, ultra-early tranexamic acid (administered as 1 g IV bolus followed by continuous infusion of 1 g every 8 hours until aneurysm treatment or 24 hours after initiation of treatment) was administered to 480 patients and compared to 475 controls.[12] The study did not show statistically significant differences in rebleeding rates between the two groups (10% in the tranexamic acid group, 14% in the control group). A good outcome (defined as a modified Rankin score 0–3) at 6 months was observed in 60% of patients in the tranexamic group versus 64% of controls, and an excellent outcome (defined as a modified Rankin score 0–2) was less frequent in the tranexamic acid group. There were no differences between the two groups in the incidence of serious adverse events. Based on this study, antifibrinolytic drugs are no longer recommended in the acute management of the patient with SAH.[2,3]

among members of a multidisciplinary team. The decision should be individualized based on patient- and aneurysm-related characteristics in the context of local logistics and expertise. Open microsurgery should be considered in younger individuals, especially in those with anterior circulation aneurysms and good clinical grade.[19] Younger patients have many years of life expectancy, and they are more likely to benefit from the more durable microsurgical clipping. Younger patients in good clinical condition (World Federation of Neurosurgical Societies [WFNS] grades 1–3) also tend to tolerate surgery better than older patients and those with higher grade SAH. After observing over the years, a handful of delayed rebleeding cases in noncompliant patients who did not follow up after endovascular treatment of their ruptured aneurysm, we have also extended a microsurgery first policy to patients who have a history of noncompliance with medical recommendations. In all other circumstances, when equipoise exists, the evidence indicates that endovascular therapy is associated with better functional results at the expense of lower rates of complete occlusion, requiring close long-term follow-up and possibly retreatment.[20]

TREATMENT OF HYDROCEPHALUS AND INCREASED INTRACRANIAL PRESSURE

Treatment of hydrocephalus in aSAH has traditionally been reserved for patients in poor neurologic condition and for those with documented dilation of the ventricular system on imaging that is associated with compromised or worsening clinical condition. However, increasing evidence suggests that ICP may be one of the most important targets to decrease secondary damage after aneurysm rupture in order to improve outcome.[21] Moreover, using ventricular size as a surrogate for increased ICP is misleading, as severely elevated ICP is present in many patients with small ventricles, especially in those with poor-grade aSAH.[22]

There is no consensus about the indication for cerebrospinal fluid (CSF) diversion after aSAH. The AHA guidelines state that "… urgent CSF diversion with external ventricular drain (EVD) and/or lumbar drain (LD) should be performed in patients with acute symptomatic hydrocephalus."[2] Nevertheless, a lot of variability persists in the practice of CSF diversion and ICP monitoring after aSAH. A subgroup analysis of Intracranial pressure monitoring in patients with acute brain injury in the intensive care unit (SYNAPSE-ICU), a multicenter, international, prospective, observational cohort study of 423 patients with aSAH from 92 units in 32 countries showed marked variability in the incidence of CSF diversion and ICP monitoring with rates ranging from 4.7% to 79.9% across different centers.[23] In this study, patients with ICP monitoring likely received more aggressive intensive therapy with a positive effect on mortality.

There is a concern that CSF diversion in the acute phase after aSAH may induce aneurysm rebleeding by suddenly decreasing transmural pressure across the aneurysm. Several studies have examined this issue, and it appears that the risk is increased in those patients with poor-grade aSAH and those with larger aneurysms.[24] In patients with such risk factors, if possible, expedited obliteration of the aneurysm should be considered while temporarily addressing ICP elevation with osmotherapy until the aneurysm is occluded and CSF diversion initiated. If CSF diversion is undertaken in a patient with an unprotected aneurysm, it is important to avoid draining CSF during catheter placement. Once the intrathecal catheter is placed, it should be set at a level high enough to avoid rapid pressure changes across the walls of the unprotected aneurysm. One should consider that the ventricular system is initially highly compliant, especially in young individuals, and can accommodate relatively large increments of pressure with only minimal changes in its caliber. Therefore, a significant reduction in ICP can be achieved with draining just a few drops of CSF.

While CSF diversion has been traditionally achieved through the utilization of an EVD, over the past 20 years there has been an increasing interest in obtaining CSF diversion through an LD instead. Since no transgression of brain parenchyma is required with LD placement, brain trauma is avoided and there is no risk of intracranial hemorrhage. In addition, there is a theoretical advantage from draining bloody CSF from the lumbar subarachnoid space rather than the ventricles since that would achieve more effective clearing of subarachnoid blood, potentially decreasing the severity of vasospasm which is secondary, for the most part, to the effects of oxyhemoglobin and its degradation products.

Following a single-center series,[25] recent randomized trials on the effects of an LD in aSAH have been completed.[26,27] Al-Tamimi and coworkers conducted a single-center, prospective, randomized controlled trial comparing LD + standard care with standard care alone. Each study group contained 105 patients treated between 2006 and 2010. The addition of an LD to standard care resulted in significantly lower incidences of neurologic deficits secondary to delayed cerebral ischemia (DCI) without a significant effect on outcome at 6 months. Major limitations of this study included its single-center nature and enrollment of good grade patients only (WFNS grades 1–3) which may have rendered the study insufficiently powered to show meaningful differences in outcome.[26]

Recently, the EARLYDRAIN investigators reported their findings in a multicenter, parallel-group, randomized controlled trial conducted between 2011 and 2016 at 19 centers across Germany, Switzerland, and Canada.[27] Patients with good and high-grade SAH were enrolled and randomized to one of two groups: 144 patients received an LD (and standard care), 143 received standard care only. Lumbar drainage was started within 72 hours of aSAH. Of note, 71% of patients in the LD group had a concomitant EVD. Despite the amount of CSF drained over the first week being similar in both groups, patients in the LD group had significantly lower ICP values suggesting that an LD was more efficient in attenuating ICP. An unfavorable outcome at 6 months occurred in 32.6% of patients in the LD group and 44.8% receiving standard care alone. Interestingly, there was no difference between groups in the frequency of vasospasm diagnosed clinically by transcranial Doppler ultrasonography or catheter angiography. Despite no differences in vasospasm incidence on imaging, 39.9% of patients in the standard care group experienced a secondary infarction on the last cerebral imaging compared to 28.5% in the LD group. The observation that the vasospasm rate was not different but that DCI infarcts were significantly lower in the LD group (in whom ICP was more effectively controlled) suggests the critical importance of controlling ICP, especially in the period after aSAH when the risk for vasospasm and secondary injury is higher. Indeed, mounting evidence suggests that ICP modulation with aggressive CSF diversion may play a critically important role in mitigating the effects of the aSAH itself and delayed vasospasm, thus improving outcomes after aSAH.

Eighty-one percent of patients undergoing continuous ICP monitoring after aSAH experience at least one episode of ICP greater than 20 mm Hg lasting at least 5 minutes.[28] Elevated ICP may reduce perfusion pressure which can have deleterious effects especially in the presence of vasospasm. Very high cerebral perfusion pressure (>100 mm Hg) is associated with better outcomes after SAH.[29]

Traditionally, threshold ICP values for patients with SAH have been extrapolated from weak evidence gathered in patients with a completely different pathologic process: head injury. Increasing evidence suggests that ICP values considered acceptable in patients with head injuries may be detrimental in the setting of SAH. Fugate and coworkers reported an illustrative case of a patient admitted with aSAH complicated by hydrocephalus.[30] The patient underwent treatment of the aneurysm and placement of an EVD which was maintained continuously opened at 15 mm Hg. Seventy-two hours after admission, the patient's condition deteriorated, and a CT perfusion showed hypoperfusion in the watershed zones. Lowering the EVD to 5 resulted in resolution of the hypoperfused areas and marked clinical improvement of the patient. In line with this observation, Samuelsson and coworkers monitored brain metabolites in 33 patients with SAH using microdialysis.[31] They found that a favorable metabolic profile was associated with values of ICP less than 10 mm Hg. Similarly, Cagnazzo and colleagues conducted a prospective study in consecutive patients with aSAH undergoing coiling and requiring EVD.[32] They observed that ICP lower than 6.7 mm Hg was beneficial in lowering the risk of DCI-related infarction. Mean ICP values among patients developing DCI-related cerebral infarction was 11 mm Hg compared to 6 mm Hg in those without ischemic lesions. They suggested that controlling ICP to very low values decreases transmural pressure across microvessels at the level of the microcirculation, thus lessening the risk of tissue ischemia from vasospasm.

In line with these observations, for several years, we have adopted a very aggressive stance with correction of ICP to very low levels by maintaining continuous CSF drainage in most patients with aSAH throughout the entire period of DCI risk. In addition, as explained later, we have a very low threshold to shunt. Our impression is that such a policy has resulted in better cognitive outcomes and a return to premorbid condition for most patients admitted in good grade (WFNS grades 1–3) and those grade 4 patients who improve to a lower grade after ICP correction. We think that this specific concept should be a main focus of future aSAH research because of its very important therapeutic implications. Additional benefits of prompt and aggressive correction of ICP in patients with aSAH include resolution of systemic hypertension (except in those with refractory/previously untreated hypertension), resolution of stress-induced hyperglycemia, and improvement in the severity of headache.

Another aspect which deserves further investigation is the identification of those patients who benefit from conversion of an EVD or LD to a permanent ventriculoperitoneal (VP) shunt. The availability of modern programmable valves and neuronavigation to place ventricular catheters has greatly decreased the immediate and late morbidity and complications related to VP shunting in patients with aSAH. Much has been written on the best protocol (slow vs rapid wean of ventricular catheters) to select patients who need VP shunting, yet no valid conclusion has been reached.[33] However, current methods to select appropriate patients are rather simplistic and rely on clinical worsening and/or ventricular system enlargement, while the EVD is weaned or clamped. Such practice exposes the patient to the risk of intracranial hypertension, which can still be deleterious in the later phase of aSAH. More research is needed to devise atraumatic methods to precisely select those patients who need VP shunting. Convinced that even the slightest communicating hydrocephalus can have deleterious effects on the cognitive and psychological recovery of these patients, "when in doubt, we shunt." This practice has been reinforced by repeated experiences of patients in whom the EVD was removed in the intensive care unit, but then VP shunting was required within a month due to suboptimal clinical recovery. This change of course highlights the crucial importance of diligent follow-up of these patients after discharge.

PREVENTION AND TREATMENT OF VASOSPASM

Vasospasm is a very common complication of SAH and likely represents the phylogenetic response to extravasation of blood out of the arterial tree and a defensive mechanism to decrease further blood loss. After a phase of acute spasm at the time of rupture (which probably happens more frequently than diagnosed on imaging), delayed vasospasm develops over time, reaching a peak between days 4 and 10 after the original bleed. Because of this delay, vasospasm offers a potential target for therapeutic intervention.

Over the past 40 years, many pharmacologic and interventional treatments have been studied with only oral nimodipine showing positive results in trials conducted 3 decades ago. Multiple studies, such as the recent trials evaluating the endothelin antagonist clazosentan, have shown that even when radiological vasospasm was prevented, functional outcome was not improved. Because of this, we and others believe that it is time to look at this phenomenon from a different viewpoint and move away from the fixation of preventing angiographic vasospasm. Likely, patients during the vasospasm risk period are at high risk for secondary injury from other neurologic (eg, increased ICP, decreased perfusion pressure) and medical complications. Therefore, once the aneurysm is secured and ICP is controlled, it is important to respect a minimalistic approach and avoid any changes which could compromise cerebral perfusion (such as hypovolemia and premature EVD weaning) until the patient is over the period of ischemic risk.

Monitoring of DCI is mostly a clinical task, though serial transcranial Doppler, continuous electroencephalography, and especially CT angiography and CT perfusion may be useful in patients with a confounded neurologic examination. We reserve catheter angiography to situations in which endovascular therapy will be necessary. Other invasive diagnostic techniques, such as brain tissue oxygen monitoring, may be helpful in comatose patients.

When patients develop signs of DCI, blood pressure augmentation (typically using norepinephrine infusion) is our first-line therapy. The addition of IV milrinone can be useful both as an inotrope and a cerebral vasodilator, but it should be used while cautiously avoiding any rapid drop in systemic blood pressure. When these interventions fail, prompt endovascular therapy is indicated. While the effects of angioplasty are more durable, vasospasm is typically diffuse and predominantly affects distal arteries. Thus, intra-arterial infusion of vasodilators (calcium channel blockers or milrinone) is most frequently used. While none of these therapeutic modalities are supported by solid evidence from randomized studies, they are broadly considered effective in practice, and consequently, there is no equipoise for randomization into trials comparing them against placebo.

MEDICAL COMPLICATIONS

A myriad of systemic complications can occur during the acute phase of aSAH in the intensive care unit. During the first 24 to 48 hours, cardiac failure, arrhythmias, and respiratory failure (from pulmonary edema, aspiration pneumonia, or atelectasis) are most threatening. Most cases of cardiac failure are caused by stress-induced cardiomyopathy from neurocardiogenic injury triggered by the massive release of catecholamines into the circulation at the time of aneurysm rupture. On echocardiogram, its most characteristic presentation is apical ballooning.[34] Contractile myocardial function can be severely reduced during the first few days but typically recovers well over the ensuing weeks. Pulmonary edema can result from neurogenic or cardiogenic mechanisms. Positive pressure ventilation, most often combined with diuretics, generally improves lung edema very effectively.

Later in the course of aSAH, hyponatremia (from cerebral salt wasting and, to a lesser degree, excessive secretion of antidiuretic hormone), central fever, infections, and venous thrombosis can develop. Because hyponatremia is caused by primary diuresis leading to polyuria, and the excessive fluid loss can cause intravascular volume contraction, it is crucial to replace salt and fluids.[35] However, inducing a positive fluid balance is not necessary and, in fact, it can be detrimental and should be avoided.[36] Fludrocortisone can reduce natriuresis, when this medication is prescribed, potassium replacement is required to correct increased urinary loss of this electrolyte.

DISCLOSURE

G. Lanzino is a consultant for Nested Knowledge and Superior Medical Editors.

REFERENCES

1. Rabinstein AA, Lanzino G, Wijdicks EF. Multidisciplinary management and emerging therapeutic strategies in aneurysmal subarachnoid haemorrhage. Lancet Neurol 2010;9(5):504–19.
2. Hoh BL, Ko NU, Amin-Hanjani S, et al. 2023 guideline for the management of patients with aneurysmal subarachnoid hemorrhage: a guideline from the American Heart Association/American Stroke Association. Stroke 2023;54(7):e314–70.
3. Treggiari MM, Rabinstein AA, Busl KM, et al. Guidelines for the neurocritical care management of aneurysmal subarachnoid hemorrhage. Neurocritical Care 2023; 39(1):1–28.
4. Molenberg R, Aalbers MW, Appelman APA, et al. Intracranial aneurysm wall enhancement as an indicator of instability: a systematic review and meta-analysis. Eur J Neurol 2021;28(11):3837–48.
5. Karamchandani RR, Fletcher JJ, Pandey AS, et al. Incidence of delayed seizures, delayed cerebral ischemia and poor outcome with the use of levetiracetam versus phenytoin after aneurysmal subarachnoid hemorrhage. J Clin Neurosci 2014;21(9):1507–13.
6. Naidech AM, Kreiter KT, Janjua N, et al. Phenytoin exposure is associated with functional and cognitive disability after subarachnoid hemorrhage. Stroke 2005; 36(3):583–7.
7. Lu VM, Graffeo CS, Perry A, et al. Rebleeding drives poor outcome in aneurysmal subarachnoid hemorrhage independent of delayed cerebral ischemia: a propensity-score matched cohort study. J Neurosurg 2019;1–9.
8. Linzey JR, Williamson C, Rajajee V, et al. Twenty-four-hour emergency intervention versus early intervention in aneurysmal subarachnoid hemorrhage. J Neurosurg 2018;128(5):1297–303.
9. Rawal S, Alcaide-Leon P, Macdonald RL, et al. Meta-analysis of timing of endovascular aneurysm treatment in subarachnoid haemorrhage: inconsistent results of early treatment within 1 day. J Neurol Neurosurg Psychiatry 2017;88(3):241–8.
10. Lanzino G, Kassell NF. Surgical treatment of the ruptured aneurysm. Timing. Neurosurg Clin N Am 1998;9(3):541–8.
11. Hillman J, Fridriksson S, Nilsson O, et al. Immediate administration of tranexamic acid and reduced incidence of early rebleeding after aneurysmal subarachnoid hemorrhage: a prospective randomized study. J Neurosurg 2002;97(4):771–8.
12. Post R, Germans MR, Tjerkstra MA, et al. Ultra-early tranexamic acid after subarachnoid haemorrhage (ULTRA): a randomised controlled trial. Lancet 2021; 397(10269):112–8.
13. Molyneux A, Kerr R, Stratton I, et al. International Subarachnoid Aneurysm Trial (ISAT) of neurosurgical clipping versus endovascular coiling in 2143 patients

with ruptured intracranial aneurysms: a randomised trial. Lancet 2002;360(9342): 1267–74.

14. Molyneux AJ, Birks J, Clarke A, et al. The durability of endovascular coiling versus neurosurgical clipping of ruptured cerebral aneurysms: 18 year follow-up of the UK cohort of the International Subarachnoid Aneurysm Trial (ISAT). Lancet 2015;385(9969):691–7.

15. Molyneux AJ, Kerr RS, Birks J, et al. Risk of recurrent subarachnoid haemorrhage, death, or dependence and standardised mortality ratios after clipping or coiling of an intracranial aneurysm in the International Subarachnoid Aneurysm Trial (ISAT): long-term follow-up. Lancet Neurol 2009;8(5):427–33.

16. Raabe A, Beck J, Gerlach R, et al. Near-infrared indocyanine green video angiography: a new method for intraoperative assessment of vascular flow. Neurosurgery 2003;52(1):132–9 [discussion 139].

17. Spelle L, Herbreteau D, Caroff J, et al. CLinical Assessment of WEB device in Ruptured aneurYSms (CLARYS): results of 1-month and 1-year assessment of re-bleeding protection and clinical safety in a multicenter study. J Neurointerventional Surg 2022;14(8):807–14.

18. Giorgianni A, Agosti E, Molinaro S, et al. Flow diversion for acutely ruptured intracranial aneurysms treatment: a retrospective study and literature review. J Stroke Cerebrovasc Dis 2022;31(3):106284.

19. Mitchell P, Kerr R, Mendelow AD, et al. Could late rebleeding overturn the superiority of cranial aneurysm coil embolization over clip ligation seen in the International Subarachnoid Aneurysm Trial? J Neurosurg 2008;108(3):437–42.

20. Lanzino G, Murad MH, d'Urso PI, et al. Coil embolization versus clipping for ruptured intracranial aneurysms: a meta-analysis of prospective controlled published studies. AJNR Am J Neuroradiol 2013;34(9):1764–8.

21. Addis A, Baggiani M, Citerio G. Intracranial pressure monitoring and management in aneurysmal subarachnoid hemorrhage. Neurocritical Care 2023. https://doi.org/10.1007/s12028-023-01752-y.

22. Bailes JE, Spetzler RF, Hadley MN, et al. Management morbidity and mortality of poor-grade aneurysm patients. J Neurosurg 1990;72(4):559–66.

23. Baggiani M, Graziano F, Rebora P, et al. Intracranial pressure monitoring practice, treatment, and effect on outcome in aneurysmal subarachnoid hemorrhage. Neurocritical Care 2023;38(3):741–51.

24. Cagnazzo F, Gambacciani C, Morganti R, et al. Aneurysm rebleeding after placement of external ventricular drainage: a systematic review and meta-analysis. Acta Neurochir 2017;159(4):695–704.

25. Hulou MM, Essibayi MA, Benet A, et al. Lumbar drainage after aneurysmal subarachnoid hemorrhage: a systematic review and meta-analysis. World Neurosurg 2022;166:261–7.e269.

26. Al-Tamimi YZ, Bhargava D, Feltbower RG, et al. Lumbar drainage of cerebrospinal fluid after aneurysmal subarachnoid hemorrhage: a prospective, randomized, controlled trial (LUMAS). Stroke 2012;43(3):677–82.

27. Wolf S, Mielke D, Barner C, et al. Effectiveness of lumbar cerebrospinal fluid drain among patients with aneurysmal subarachnoid hemorrhage: a randomized clinical trial. JAMA Neurol 2023;80(8):833–42.

28. Zoerle T, Lombardo A, Colombo A, et al. Intracranial pressure after subarachnoid hemorrhage. Crit Care Med 2015;43(1):168–76.

29. Ryttlefors M, Howells T, Nilsson P, et al. Secondary insults in subarachnoid hemorrhage: occurrence and impact on outcome and clinical deterioration. Neurosurgery 2007;61(4):704–14 [discussion 714-705].

30. Fugate JE, Rabinstein AA, Wijdicks EF, et al. Aggressive CSF diversion reverses delayed cerebral ischemia in aneurysmal subarachnoid hemorrhage: a case report. Neurocritical Care 2012;17(1):112–6.
31. Samuelsson C, Howells T, Kumlien E, et al. Relationship between intracranial hemodynamics and microdialysis markers of energy metabolism and glutamate-glutamine turnover in patients with subarachnoid hemorrhage. Clinical article. J Neurosurg 2009;111(5):910–5.
32. Cagnazzo F, Chalard K, Lefevre PH, et al. Optimal intracranial pressure in patients with aneurysmal subarachnoid hemorrhage treated with coiling and requiring external ventricular drainage. Neurosurg Rev 2021;44(2):1191–204.
33. Palasz J, D'Antona L, Farrell S, et al. External ventricular drain management in subarachnoid haemorrhage: a systematic review and meta-analysis. Neurosurg Rev 2022;45(1):365–73.
34. Fujita T, Nakaoka Y, Hayashi S, et al. Incidence and clinical characteristics of takotsubo syndrome in patients with subarachnoid hemorrhage. Int Heart J 2022; 63(3):517–23.
35. Busl KM, Rabinstein AA. Prevention and correction of dysnatremia after aneurysmal subarachnoid hemorrhage. Neurocritical Care 2023;39(1):70–80.
36. Kissoon NR, Mandrekar JN, Fugate JE, et al. Positive fluid balance is associated with poor outcomes in subarachnoid hemorrhage. J Stroke Cerebrovasc Dis 2015;24(10):2245–51.

Neuroendovascular Rescue 2025
Trends in Stroke Endovascular Therapy

Camilo R. Gomez, MD, MBA*, Brandi R. French, MD,
Francisco E. Gomez, MD, Adnan I. Qureshi, MD

KEYWORDS

- Stroke • Endovascular therapy • Neuroendovascular • Neurology • Therapy
- Endovascular management

KEY POINTS

- Neuroendovascular rescue of acute ischemic stroke continues to evolve into a spectrum of techniques of variable technic complexity
- Increasingly sophisticated imaging techniques allow better patient selection geared at optimizing outcomes of neuroendovascular rescue
- The success of neuroendovascular resucue procedures is interdependent with optimal periprocedural care of these patients

INTRODUCTION

The emergent endovascular management of patients with acute ischemic stroke (AIS) caused by a large arterial occlusion (LAO) exploded following the 2015 publication of pivotal clinical trials demonstrating the consistent beneficial effect of arterial recanalization, irrespective of whether the patients had already received intravenous tissue-type plasminogen activator (IV-tPA) or not.[1] As such, the concept of *Neuroendovascular Rescue* (ie, "rescue"), introduced in the 1990s at a time when technology had not caught up with the interest of using mechanical means to restore cerebral blood flow (CBF), found evident footing to justify becoming the standard of care in the subpopulation of AIS patients with occlusion of the internal carotid (ICA) and/or middle cerebral arteries (MCA).[2] Since then, although *thrombectomy* remains the fundamental method used for arterial recanalization, technical and procedural innovations translate into increasingly complex rescue concepts and approaches. In turn, this has expanded the target population that can potentially benefit from intervention

University of Missouri Columbia School of Medicine, Columbia, MO, USA
* Corresponding author. Department of Neurology – University of Missouri, 548 CS&E Building – One Hospital Drive, Columbia, MO 65212.
E-mail address: crgomez@missouri.edu

Neurol Clin 42 (2024) 717–738
https://doi.org/10.1016/j.ncl.2024.03.006
0733-8619/24/© 2024 Elsevier Inc. All rights reserved.

to the vertebrobasilar system,[3] *not-so-large arterial occlusions* (NSLAO),[4–6] those with *in situ* causative cerebrovascular pathology,[7–12] and even to those with established infarction in a partial volume of the affected arterial territory.[13–16] The ingenuity driving the most recent advances has also uncovered the promise to expand the application of these techniques to increasingly larger subpopulations, thereby improving their ultimate clinical outcomes.

The present is a review of relevant advances made in AIS rescue, organized in the context of the state of the art, trends and outlook relative to its historical progression. We have structured our review along the following topics: (1) technical advances in endovascular arterial recanalization, (2) improvements in patient selection techniques, (3) expansion of the application of reperfusion techniques, (4) integration of adjuvant techniques for revascularization, and (5) optimization of periprocedural care.

TECHNICAL ADVANCES IN ENDOVASCULAR ARTERIAL RECANALIZATION
Evolution and State of the Art

The interest in using mechanical means to treat LAO causing AIS followed years of using intra-arterial instillation of thrombolytic agents.[2,17,18] This practice, popular in the 1980s and 1990s, carried inherent limitations such as the protracted time required for many of the embolic particles to be "cleared" by the administered pharmacologic agent, as well as the unpredictable retention of thrombolytic agent within the microcirculation, increasing the risk of delayed hemorrhagic complications. Along these lines, it is therefore not surprising that the prospective, randomized clinical trials using this technique rendered only modest evidence of clinical benefit,[19,20] resulting in failure of approval of thrombolytic agents for this indication, reduced widespread adoption of this technique, and a shift toward finding a faster and safer mechanical approach to urgent recanalization of cerebral LAO.[2]

Through the 1990s, the initial attempts at using mechanical rescue methods relied on the only technology available at that time: Snares! Although reported to be successful in different case reports and small series, the inherent difficulty of securing the 3-dimensional occluding particle using a 2-dimensional device rendered the technique unreliable and time-consuming, thereby reducing its practical and widespread application.[21–23] Shortly thereafter, the introduction of *retrievers* (ie, devices specifically designed to remove intraluminal occluding material) paved the way for the design and completion of the clinical trials that ultimately proved urgent percutaneous thrombectomy (ie, the physical extraction of an occluding thrombus/embolus) led to better outcomes in patients with AIS caused by LAO, irrespective of pretreatment with intravenous thrombolysis.[24–28] By 2015, the concerted publication of several pivotal studies, with unquestionably favorable results, created the framework for the rapid growth and development of this practice.[1]

Simultaneously, advances in the design and manufacture of distal access catheters (DACs) with increasingly soft and flexible tips, capable of being advanced directly into the first order cerebral arteries not only facilitated retriever deployment but also allowed direct clot aspiration, either manually or using a vacuum pump (**Fig. 1**).[29–32] The overlap of these two techniques led to their utilization either concurrently or synchronously to improve the resulting recanalization of the cerebral arteries. Presently, the increasing availability of smaller and more trackable DAC has resulted in faster and safer thrombectomy procedures. In addition, it has allowed operators to target occluding particles located downstream from the first order arteries, targeting NSLAO, a topic to be covered more in-depth in the following paragraphs.

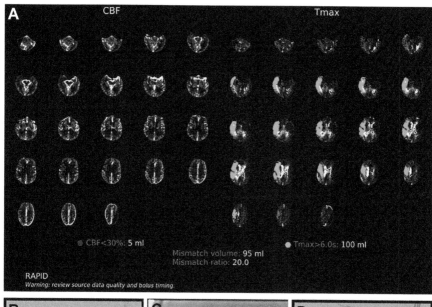

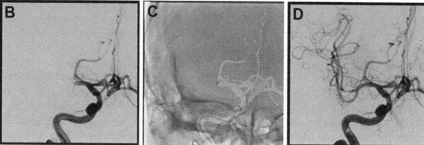

Fig. 1. Qualifying perfusion scan and rescue. (*A*) A woman presenting with an acute right middle cerebral artery occlusion and a moderate neurovascular deficit (NIHSS = 7), was found to have a type I CT perfusion scan (ie, small core [5 cc], large penumbra [100 cc] and mismatch [95 cc]). (*B*) The original angiographic images confirmed the occlusion. (*C*) She underwent direct thrombectomy with an aspiration direct access catheter. (*D*) Removal of the occlusive particle, successfully led to large arterial recanalization. NIHSS, National Institutes of Health Stroke Scale.

Future Trends and Opportunities

The current underpinning of AIS rescue is that of increasingly ultrarapid access to the occluding particle, having recognized that expedient recanalization has a significant impact on the ultimate outcome.[33] Consequently, there is a steady surge of large-bore (ie, 0.062–0.088″ inner diameter), flexible, soft-tipped (ie, tip load ≤ 1 g), aspiration DAC (ADAC) that can be advanced quickly into the first-order cerebral arteries, allowing massive aspiration and in toto removal of the occluding particle, with decreased risk of fragmentation and downstream embolization (see **Fig. 1**). In addition, ADAC modifications, such as the introduction of a beveled tip that reshapes it from circular to oval and increases the area of clot contact for aspiration, promise to improve their performance.[34,35] In parallel, retriever technology continues to advance, capitalizing on the original design of a device that can be deployed and then retrieved while dragging the occluding thrombus with it. Advances introduced in this area include separate 3-dimensional intraluminal chambers,[36] interlinked caged technology,[37] helical slits with a proximal closed ring,[38] and adjustable diameter.[39,40] Finally, similar advances in engineering are being applied to produce smaller ADAC and retrievers that allow the operators to reach vessels downstream from the first-order arteries (eg, MCA divisions and branches). This will continue to expand the applications of the technique to a larger patient population, with literature supporting its beneficial effect.[5,29,41,42]

IMPROVEMENTS IN PATIENT SELECTION TECHNIQUES
Evolution and State of the Art

In the early days of AIS rescue (ie, 1980–1990s), operators selected patients only when they presented with clinical syndromes suggestive of a LAO and their noncontrast computed tomography (NCCT) failed to show established infarction of the arterial territory of concern.[2] Over time, the introduction of imaging techniques that allowed surrogate quantification of ischemic tissue volume changed the landscape of patient selection, and even expanded the therapeutic window based on the understanding that the impact of the passage of time is neither linear nor absolute, but exponential and relative.[43] Indeed, advances in devices and operational strategies have been paralleled by improved diagnostic algorithms geared at identifying the ideal patients to benefit from urgent intervention (ie, those most likely to have an optimal functional outcome and least likely to suffer unplanned reperfusion injuries), whose composite attributes define a profile equivalent to a "high value target" (HVT).[44]

Patient selection on the basis of the difference between the volume of potentially salvageable ischemic brain tissue (ie, tissue "at risk", or "ischemic penumbra"), and tissue already infarcted and beyond any hope of recovery even by flow restoration constitutes the central concept of urgent assessment of AIS. The difference (ie, "mismatch") in volume between ischemic penumbra and infarcted tissue, is directly proportional to the opportunity for successful urgent intervention and good clinical outcomes.[43] Since smaller infarct volumes are associated with better outcomes, the larger the mismatch the better the patient qualifies as an HVT (see **Fig. 1**).[43,44] In fact, the success of contemporary thrombectomy clinical trials is largely the result of having incorporated mismatch imaging criteria for patient selection and recruitment.[44]

Presently, assessment of this mismatch can be effectively carried out using computed tomographic perfusion (CTP) scans, and relies on surrogate markers that measure delay and dispersion of flow through collateral pathways: (1) the mean transit time of the contrast through the tissue, (2) the time to peak (TTP) or raw concentration-time curve, and (3) the TTP of the deconvoluted tissue residue function (Tmax), which can then be compared with volumes of tissue infarcted or with high probability of being infarcted (ie, ischemic "core"; **Figs. 2** and **3**). Although NCCT is capable of demonstrating infarcted tissue, it does not perform optimally in the early interval of the ischemic process, even when incorporating paradigms such as the Alberta Stroke Program Early CT Score (ASPECTS). Therefore, assessing the volume of tissue with the deepest degree of ischemia (ie, ischemic "core") by quantifying CBF or cerebral blood volume correlates and commonly predicts final infarct volume in the context of no reperfusion (see **Figs. 1–3**). Alternatively, various MRI sequences can also be utilized for patient selection and HVT identification. In this context, volume of infarcted tissue is best accomplished by using fluid attenuated inversion recovery sequences,

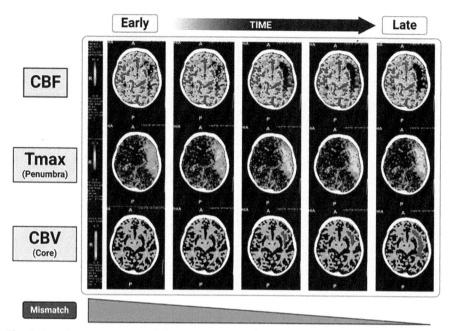

Fig. 2. Imaging surrogates and time progression of ischemia. Following arterial occlusion, tissue ischemia progressively evolves over time, following a centrifugal path, resulting in steady expansion of the ischemic core and concurrent reduction of the mismatch between this and the overall ischemic volume. Persistence of the occlusion results in permanent ischemic injury of the volume affected (Created with BioRender.com.). CBF, cerebral blood flow; Tmax, time to peak of the deconvoluted tissue residue function; CBV, cerebral blood volume.

while diffusion-weighted imaging (DWI) MRI allows very early detection of ischemic brain tissue (ie, not necessarily infarcted). This attribute makes DWI very attractive for early estimation measurements when combined with perfusion-weighted MRI surrogates, which are similar to those used in CTP. Irrespective of which technique is used, assessment of penumbra versus core mismatch by comparing different surrogates has become the standard of care in the identification of patients with HVT for urgent intervention.

In practice, the emergent assessment of patients with AIS based on these principles leads to 1 of 4 potential types of perfusion maps, characterized by the qualitative magnitudes of ischemic core and ischemic mismatch (see **Fig. 3**). The thresholds originally used to dichotomize these parameters as either "small" or "large", based on the existing literature, were an absolute volume 70 cc for the ischemic core and a mismatch ratio 1.8 or greater between the two volumes. Using this paradigm, the two extreme types have the clearest clinical implications, one optimal (type I) and the other dismal (type IV), relative to urgent intervention.[43,44] Patients displaying type I perfusion maps (see **Figs. 1** and **3**) represent the ideal HVT for urgent intervention, almost irrespective of their time of presentation relative to their estimated time of onset (ETO). In fact, patients with this type of perfusion map were deliberately selected for participation in the most important prospective series, representing a major driving force for their unmistakable success.[1] Conversely, patients with Type IV perfusion maps represent the coexistence of a large volume of a likely

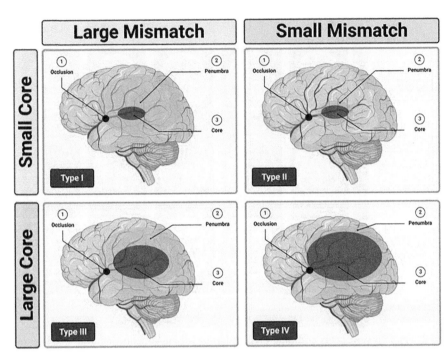

Fig. 3. Types of cerebral perfusion maps following arterial occlusion. The basis for this classification is the size of the ischemic core, and that of the mismatch between it and the overall ischemic volume (ie, the "penumbra"). In general, the smaller the core and the larger the penumbra, the better the patient qualifies for benefitting from urgent intervention. (Created with BioRender.com.).

injured tissue, concurrent with a small volume of salvageable brain must be examined more critically, since their benefit/risk ratio is materially smaller. Moreover, these patients were explicitly excluded from randomization into the major prospective retriever-based thrombectomy studies.[1] The fate of patients with types II and III perfusion maps has been somewhat more difficult to forecast but, as we discuss later, represent opportunities for expanding the benefits of endovascular interventions for AIS.

In addition to tissue ischemia assessment, computed tomographic (CT) angiography and MR angiography add the last dimension of the urgent assessment of patients with AIS with suspected LAO. Either of these techniques provides confirmation of the arterial occlusion responsible for the ischemic clinical syndrome, thereby identifying the target for intervention. In addition, given the state of the art of available devices, operators are able to evaluate details about cerebrovascular architecture and its suitability for any one of various interventional approaches available (eg, radial vs femoral arteriotomy).

Future Trends and Opportunities

Although recent publications suggest that sophisticated perfusion imaging may not be necessary, and that simply using the ASPECTS approach by NCCT is sufficient to achieve the same outcomes,[45] this constitutes an oversimplified view of the decision-making process that operators must complete before and during rescue procedures. In our opinion, abandoning the current imaging strategies described earlier in favor of simply using NCCT would be a step backwards and would lead to hindrances to future improvements in this field. So, although it is certainly *feasible* to qualify a patient for urgent intervention using NCCT, it is not *reasonable* to forego acquisition of additional relevant information likely to have significant impact in the overall care of the patient.

In general, advances in the precision of the information about cerebral perfusion and tissue viability, as well as the speed with which such information is acquired, are the driving forces that move the current trends of practice. The recognition that the identified perfusion map type simply represents a "snapshot" in the time continuum of the ischemic process has resulted in a shift to assess other more dynamic variables such as infarct growth rate (IGR).[43] The possibility of not only gauging the degree and volume of ischemia, but also the rate at which the tissue is becoming permanently injured is likely to impact various practical measures of care, such as time available for patient transport for intervention, or the application of measures of care capable of slowing down the IGR.[43]

Moreover, advances in our understanding of how to best manage patients whose perfusion map types (ie, II and III) may not have as clear a prognosis or therapeutic pathway has already begun to bear fruit, with recent literature demonstrating how neuroendovascular rescue may be beneficial for patient with type III perfusion maps (ie, "large core").[13,15,16,46] These results, however, have been somewhat predictable when considering the common mistake of equating the ischemic core with established infarction when, in fact, it only represents the volume of deepest degree of ischemia.[47–50] Thus, particularly during the early stages of the ischemic process, and combined with a normal NCCT, it must not be interpreted as permanently injured tissue, as it displays some reversibility following early therapeutic reperfusion.[47]

Conversely, patients with type II perfusion maps usually present with minimal clinical symptomatology (ie, low National Institutes of Health Stroke Scale score), have an evident LAO, and display an "exuberant" collateral circulation.[51–53] However, their risk of the ischemic process worsening, with consequent clinical deterioration has been identified, and the most recent literature favors proceeding with intervention, even within very protracted therapeutic windows.[54–57]

Presently, most institutions utilize computerized algorithms via dedicated imaging analysis software to expedite ischemic tissue calculations, ASPECTS analysis, and LAO assessments, notably RapidAI (iSchemaView, Inc San Mateo, CA; see **Fig. 1**) and Viz.AI (Viz.AI, Inc San Francisco, CA), both of which incorporate artificial intelligence into their algorithms. Despite their reliability continuing to improve, it is unlikely that they will completely replace the expert human factor. That said, they will progressively incorporate more precise information which, in turn, should result in better diagnostic and therapeutic decisions.

EXPANSION OF THE APPLICATION OF REPERFUSION TECHNIQUES
Evolution and State of the Art

Historically, the introduction of neuroendovascular rescue by any means began by targeting patients who presented with AIS due to LAO. From the interventional point of view, such a focused application followed important considerations of reasonableness and feasibility: (1) LAO typically resulted in easily recognizable and characteristic stroke syndromes, with severe neurologic deficits and high mortality; (2) target occluded arteries were of sufficient caliber to allow procedural completion using the available devices at the time; and (3) the occlusive clot burdens were so large that exclusive treatment with IV-tPA proved to be insufficient to assure recanalization. In this context, 2 specific clinical scenarios were considered of primary importance in the application of urgent endovascular techniques for AIS: (1) occlusion of the ICA and/or trunk of the MCA and (2) occlusion of the basilar artery.

Over the years, a number of series reported improved outcomes using intra-arterial thrombolytic agents (ie, urokinase, pro-urokinase, alteplase, tenecteplase, reteplase) to recanalize the first-order arteries in the carotid and vertebrobasilar circulations.[17–20] However, following the 2015 publication of several pivotal clinical trials, thrombectomy was quickly adopted as the primary therapeutic consideration in patients with occlusion of the ICA or MCA.[1] Since then, numerous other publications have introduced varied techniques and different devices for revascularization, while still concentrating in the carotid circulation. More recently, publications demonstrating the success of neuroendovascular rescue in the vertebrobasilar system have become available, immediately supporting its use to treat this patient population.[3]

In parallel to the technical advances and introduction of new devices, all of these clinical trials have shown that the effective therapeutic window for revascularization is longer than first understood.[43] As a result, the application of these procedures is no longer strictly dependent on the ischemic interval (ie, time from the ETO) but more so on the critical assessment of the ischemic penumbra mismatch described earlier, and therapeutic windows of up to 24 hours are an acceptable component of the state of the art.[1,43]

Future Trends and Opportunities

We continue to experience a rapid evolution in our ability to complete rescue procedures under more focused cerebrovascular scenarios, shifting the entire field closer to precision medicine. Smaller large bore catheters with internal diameters of 0.035 to 0.045″, as well as larger guidewires with exceedingly soft tips that allow their safe navigation intracranially, continue to be introduced, allowing operators to successfully recanalized increasingly smaller arterial branches (ie, NSLAO). The importance of this evolution is considerable, both as a primary technique to recanalize smaller arteries whose occlusion can lead to disabling deficits, or as a secondary application following recanalizing of a LAO accompanied by clot fragmentation and downstream embolization (**Fig. 4**).

In addition to device improvements, as mentioned earlier, there is now robust evidence that even those patients with type III perfusion maps, by definition having a large ischemic core, also benefit from rescue.[54–57] Again, this is not surprising considering how the ischemic core is assessed, quantified, and interpreted. The combination of a realistic interpretation of the ischemic core in the early stages of ischemia, with the ability to rapidly and safely navigate NSLAO, has expanded the population that benefits from neuroendovascular rescue.

INTEGRATION OF ADJUVANT TECHNIQUES FOR REVASCULARIZATION
Evolution and State of the Art

In the mid-1990s, concurrently with the shift from the interest in intra-arterial thrombolysis to direct thrombectomy, IV-tPA was adopted for the management of AIS.[58] Notwithstanding the controversy about the impact of preprocedural treatment with IV-tPA,[59,60] such an approach continues to represent the standard of care.[61] In parallel, percutaneous transluminal angioplasty and stenting (PTAS) of atherosclerotic

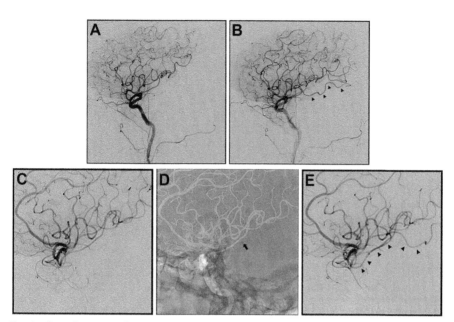

Fig. 4. Thrombectomy of an NSLAO lateral angiographic views of a patient presenting with disabling language abnormalities stemming from acute occlusion of the left parieto-occipital branch of the middle cerebral artery. Wide angled view of the left internal carotid artery injection before (*A*) and after (*B*) thrombectomy. The recanalized artery is denoted by arrowheads. Magnified working view before (*C*), during, (*D*) and after (*E*) recanalization of the target artery. The tip of a 0.043″ direct aspiration catheter if denoted by the arrow in (*D*), and the recanalized artery by the arrowheads in (*E*).

lesions of the extra and intracranial segments of the cerebral circulation continued to be developed and applied. Not surprisingly, increasingly complex neuroendovascular rescue procedures incorporate PTAS in addition to simple thrombectomy, thereby addressing the underlying causative lesion resulting in the index AIS (**Fig. 5**).[7,10,11] Clearly, more mature, and well-accepted procedures such as PTAS of the extracranial carotid contrast with PTAS of intracranial arteries, a subject of considerable controversy in the past. Still, the increasingly available body of literature suggests that concurrent use of these techniques during AIS rescue is beneficial and generally safe.[7,10,11]

Future Trends and Opportunities

Evidence of the benefit of concurrent PTAS of the extracranial carotid artery that caused downstream LAO continues to accumulate.[7] In our view, the most reasonable approach to these cases involves balloon angioplasty of the carotid lesion, followed by downstream thrombectomy of the embolic particle, and finishing with stent deployment in the carotid artery as the last step of the procedure (ie, "on the way out"; see **Fig. 5**). However, at least in some cases, the carotid artery occlusion is accompanied by significant clot burden in its cervical segment. In order to avoid additional downstream embolization, we have found the use of rheolytic thrombectomy catheters (AngioJet. Boston Scientific, Inc Marlborough, MA) to provide a practical step when incorporated in our rescue procedures, prior to completely restoring proximal flow.[62]

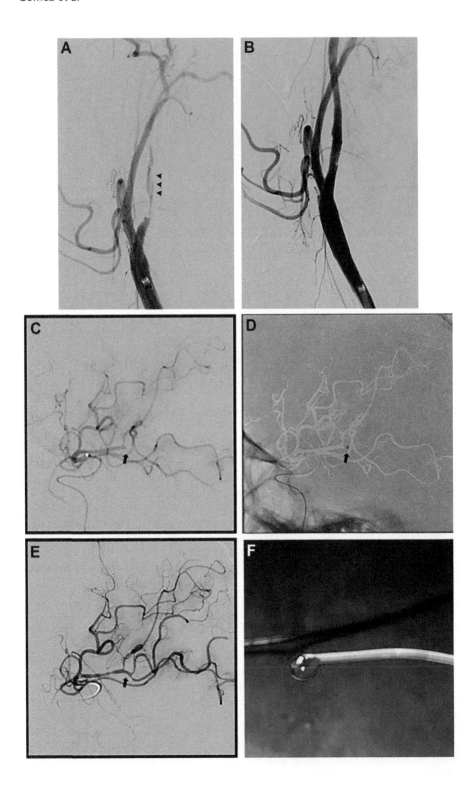

The benefit of concurrent PTAS of intracranial lesions during rescue procedures is somewhat more difficult to assess, particularly because of the heterogeneity of the pathology.[10,11] In and of itself, this attribute makes it also difficult to design prospective clinical trials without variability bias into their outcome analysis. Nevertheless, the literature continues to support the use of adjuvant PTAS, particularly in view of the significant incidence of lesion recoil with inherent risk of reocclusion.[10,11] These concepts underscore the fact that, presently, it is no longer sufficient to equate rescue with simple thrombectomy, and we must acknowledge different levels of interventional complexity (**Table 1**).

OPTIMIZATION OF PERIPROCEDURAL CARE
Evolution and State of the Art

In addition to the inherent complexity and sophistication of rescue techniques for the treatment of AIS, the periprocedural care of these patients impacts their outcome, incorporating strategies with specific objectives before, during, and after intervention (**Fig. 6**).[63] The hemodynamic management of these patients until the moment the target vessel is recanalized centers on cerebral perfusion pressure (CPP) optimization via the leptomeningeal collaterals system in support of the ischemic penumbra.[63] Throughout the interval that precedes reperfusion, the brain of patients with AIS is composed of 2 neighboring "compartments", each with own specific hemodynamic needs (**Fig. 7A**): the nonischemic normal brain tissue (ie, compartment A, not directly affected by the ictus) and the symptomatic ischemic tissue volume (ie, compartment B). The former typically maintains normal autoregulation, with CBF remaining *pressure-independent*, while the latter fails to autoregulate and is characterized by *pressure-dependent* CBF (see **Fig. 7A**). Such a "2-compartment" model leads us to manage compartment B as the primary target of collateral support, while avoiding any measures that may compromise compartment A. Pathophysiologically, compartment B constitutes a microenvironment hemodynamically homologous to "local shock". That is, as CPP and CBF drop, reducing tissue oxygen delivery (DO_2), a compensatory rise in oxygen extraction fraction (OEF) maintains tissue oxygen uptake (Vo_2) within normal levels, but only to a point. Once OEF is maximal, no longer capable of compensating, Vo_2 drops precipitously, indicating the beginning of ischemic tissue injury (**Fig. 7B**). Thus, the overall hemodynamic objective is to shift tissue perfusion from the pressure-dependent to the pressure-independent state (see **Fig. 7B**).[63]

◄───

Fig. 5. Thrombectomy PLUS carotid stenting. Lateral angiographic views of a patient presenting with acute ischemia in the posterior portion of the left hemisphere, downstream from a nearly occluded cervical internal carotid artery. (*A*) Left common carotid artery injection demonstrates near occlusion of the proximal left internal carotid artery, with a suggestion of intraluminal thrombus (*arrowheads*). (*B*) Final control left common carotid artery injection following angioplasty and stenting, demonstrating correction of the original stenotic lesion, optimal contrast opacification of the cervical segment of the left internal carotid artery and no residual intraluminal thrombus. (*C*) Left internal carotid artery injection following angioplasty of the proximal lesion, with flow restoration demonstrates downstream occlusion of the left temporal occipital segment of the inferior division of the middle cerebral artery is evident (*arrow*). (*D*) A 0.043″ distal access catheter has been advanced to the point of arterial occlusion (*arrow*) for direct aspiration thrombectomy. (*E*) Control injection of the left internal carotid artery following removal of the aspiration catheter demonstrates recanalization of the occluded cortical branch (*arrow*). (*F*) The occluding thrombus fragment was recovered directly at the tip of the aspiration catheter.

Table 1
Different levels of interventional complexity in stroke rescue

	High Value Target Attributes		
Procedural Complexity	Clinical Syndrome	Ischemic Mismatch	Large Arterial Occlusion
Category 1 Simple Thrombectomy	NIHSS ↑↑↑ (ie, >15)	CTP Types I or II (III?!)	MCA, ICA(t), ACA(i), PCA, BA, VA(i)
	COMMENTS: Minimal operational complexity and straight forward procedural blueprint. Generally, a quick procedure, with small risk, and standard of care.		
Category 2 NSLAO Thrombectomy	NIHSS ↑ or ↑↑ (ie, 6–14)	CTP Type I (Penumbra ≥ 70 mL)	MCA 2nd–3rd Order Branches
	COMMENTS: Somewhat lower benefit/risk ratio since target vessel is smaller. Operational completion can be quick. Literature favors intervention.		
Category 3 Thrombectomy PLUS	NIHSS ↑↑↑ (ie, >15)	CTP Types I or II (III?!)	Underlying or tandem stenosis
	COMMENTS: Operational complexity can be considerable, and completion is typically prolonged by the need to address the concurrent pathology. The supporting literature is limited yet favorable.		

Abbreviation: ACA, anterior cerebral artery; BA, basilar artery; CTP, computed tomography perfusion; ICA, Internal carotid artery; MCA, middle cerebral artery; NIHSS, National Institutes of Health Stroke Scale; NSLAO, Not-so-large arterial occlusion; PCA, posterior cerebral artery; VA, vertebral artery.

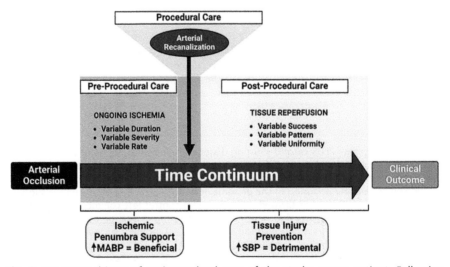

Fig. 6. Important drivers of periprocedural care of the stroke rescue patient. Following acute arterial occlusion, and along the time continuum, the care of the stroke rescue patient is substantially different before and after arterial recanalization. The entire preprocedural care is driven by maintenance of the viability of the ischemic penumbra via hemodynamic support. Following recanalization, however, prevention of tissue reperfusion injury becomes the most important driving force to the management strategy. (Created with BioRender.com.).

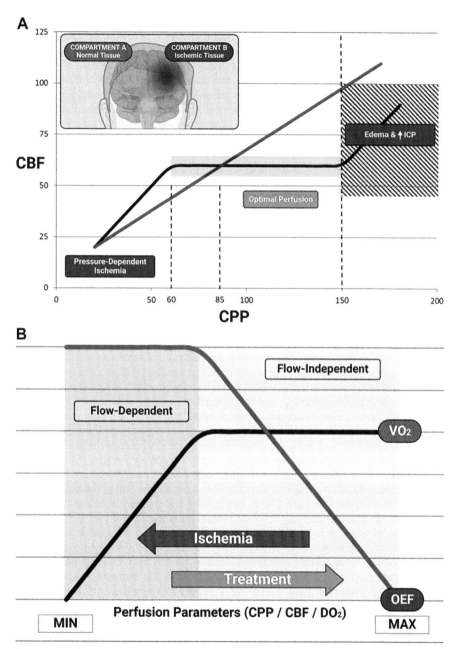

Fig. 7. Hemodynamic attributes of the brain of stroke patients: (A) "Two-Compartment" Model. Compartment A represents the normal tissue not affected by the ictus. Generally, with preserved the capacity to autoregulate blood flow within a certain range of CPP (ie, 60–150 mm Hg). Compartment B represents the ischemic tissue, which loses its capacity to autoregulate blood flow, becoming directly proportional to the CPP. The literature has consistently shown poor outcomes when cerebral perfusion pressure drops below a threshold that approximates 80 to 90 mm Hg unless reperfusion is established. (B) Ischemic Tissue "Local Shock" Physiology. As tissue perfusion decreases (ie, CPP, CBF, or DO$_2$), OEF

In this context, and just like in patients with systemic shock, periprocedural intravascular volume management is of paramount importance. The literature supports the notion that intravascular volume expansion improves leptomeningeal collaterals, and this may be more beneficial than has been previously recognized.[51,64] Moreover, dehydrated patients (ie, with low intravascular volume) are more likely to become hypotensive during the rescue procedure, thereby actively aggravating the ischemic process. Another simple care tactic during the preprocedural interval is that of managing patients with AIS in a supine and horizontal posture (ie, just like systemic shock), since this maximizes overall cardiovascular performance and CPP support. In addition, preprocedural blood pressure management must parallel that of intravascular volume in terms of following 2 clear and defined goals: primary optimization of mean arterial blood pressure (MABP), the driver of CPP, and secondary avoidance of exaggerated rises in systolic blood pressure (SBP) that increase the risk of reperfusion injury and end-organ complications. The relationship between admission blood pressure and outcomes follows a "U-shaped" curve and blood pressure extremes must not to be ignored. Based on the existing literature, the most reasonable approach is to actively reduce the SBP to less than 200 mm Hg (185 mm Hg if the patient received IV-tPA) *so long* as the MABP can be maintained no less than 100 mm Hg. This combination of variables assures that the CPP is not compromised unnecessarily, while the danger of reperfusion injury is minimized.

Procedurally, one important controversy has been whether rescue should be completed under general anesthesia. The main concern has been the frequent drops in systemic blood pressure that accompanied induction of anesthesia and which, prior to recanalization, compromise collateral support of the CPP.[52] Since this is a tangible target for process improvement,[53] most operators favor using general anesthesia for rescue procedures.[52] Curiously, recent publications suggest that some of the anesthetic agents may have neuroprotective effects that could be beneficial for AIS outcomes.[65]

Once the operator successfully completes the rescue procedure, with arterial flow restoration to an optimal level (ie, thrombolysis in cerebral infarction [TICI] = 2b or 3), systemic blood pressure should be immediately reduced to more acceptable levels, following the same strategy set forth but resetting the target values, as follow: (1) for complete reperfusion (TICI = 3) target SBP 160 mm Hg or lesser and MABP 85 mm Hg or greater, and (2) for incomplete reperfusion (TICI < 3) target SBP 170 mm Hg or lesser and MABP 90 mm Hg or greater. It is imperative that neither of the 2 components of systemic blood pressure is considered in the absence of the other. Close collaboration with anesthesiology and critical care teams to assure that the systemic blood pressure is maintained within the expected parameters is an exceedingly important task within the workflow of managing AIS patients with LAO.[53] Clear protocols, agreed upon a priori, are bound to have a beneficial impact on the overall outcome of both the procedure and the patient.

---

progressively increases as a compensatory mechanism to maintain Vo₂ leveled. At a point beyond which OEF can no longer increase and compensate, Vo₂ precipitously drops, and the tissue begins to develop permanent injury. Prioritizing improved perfusion drives all treatment strategies. (Created with BioRender.com.). CPP, cerebral perfusion pressure; CBF, cerebral blood flow; DO₂, tissue oxygen delivery; Vo₂, tissue oxygen uptake; OEF, oxygen extraction fraction.

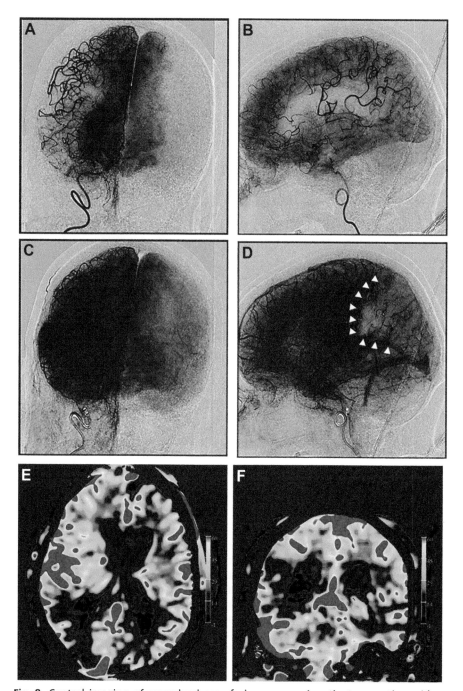

Fig. 8. Control imaging of procedural reperfusion success. A patient presenting with an acute right middle cerebral artery occlusion underwent successful (TICI = 2b) direct aspiration thrombectomy. (*A–D*) *Digital parenchymography.* Increasing the contrast and decreasing the brightness of the arteriolar–capillary phase of a conventional angiographic run allows qualitative assessment of the microcirculatory perfusion. Moreover, it allows direct comparison before (*A, B*) and after (*C, D*) intervention. In this case, it demonstrated

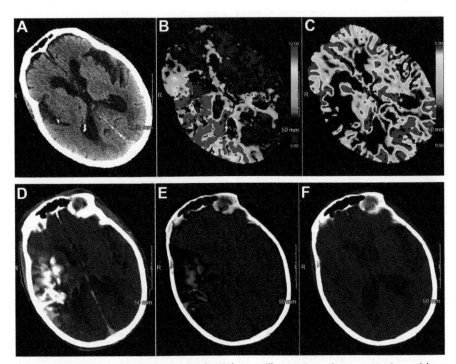

Fig. 9. Postprocedural dual energy CT (DECT) surveillance. A patient presenting with an acute right middle cerebral artery occlusion underwent successful thrombectomy, followed by immediate DECT on her way to the neurointensive care unit. (*A–C*) Preprocedurally, the patient displayed relatively normal NCCT (*A*), and a significant volume of increased Tmax (*B*), decreased CBV (*C*), and small mismatch (type III map). (*D-F*) Postprocedurally, the DECT demonstrated contrast trapping within the volume corresponding to the ischemic core assessed prior to intervention (*C*). The basic NCCT at 80 kV (*D*) demonstrated hyperdensity within this volume of tissue, fairly matched by the iodine overlay (*E*). As a result, the virtual noncontrast images (*F*) showed minimal evidence of hypodensity, indicating the findings to be related to contrast administration rather than hemorrhagic changes.

Trends and Opportunities

In addition to using conventional digital subtraction angiography to assess the magnitude and success of reperfusion at the conclusion of the procedure, additional imaging techniques amplify the scope of this task. Digital *parenchymography*, a simple postprocessing technique applicable to any angiographic run, allows immediate assessment of tissue perfusion without the need for additional contrast or radiation (**Fig. 8**).[66] More recently, cone-beam parenchymal blood volume CT imaging has become available with certain angiographic units, allowing 3-dimensional, color-graded, cerebral perfusion assessment prior to completing the procedure, without

---

residual occlusion of the right angular artery (*D, arrowheads*). (*E* and *F*) *Parenchymal blood volume CT scan.* Axial (*E*) and coronal (*F*) planes of the parenchymal blood volume cone-beam CT scan obtained following recanalization of the right middle cerebral artery, also demonstrating a perfusion defect corresponding to the right angular artery territory. CT, computed tomography.

taking the patient off the table (see **Fig. 8**).[67] We have found both of these to be useful in assessing the presence of "pockets" of tissue affected by *no-reflow phenomenon*, corresponding to recalcitrant perfusion abnormalities of the microcirculation, and which require attention in and of themselves.[68–70]

Another opportunity for using technology to facilitate postprocedural care involves dual-energy CT (DECT) surveillance scanning.[71] Historically, NCCT studies following endovascular intervention have commonly demonstrated hyperdense changes representing either hemorrhagic changes, contrast trapped in the microcirculation, or both (in addition of course to any infarcted tissue). The literature affirms that hemorrhagic changes can have a negative impact on outcome, while contrast trapped in the microcirculation does not seem to do so. Therefore, DECT is the ideal tool for rescue patients during the hours that follow the procedure, allowing some degree of differentiation between contrast and hemorrhagic changes (**Fig. 9**). Based upon the complexity and duration of the intervention, as well as the overall timeline of treatment for any particular patient, the DECT can be scheduled for a specific time after procedural completion. The results greatly assist with managing antithrombotic agents, interpreting neurologic changes, and following up on those patients who received either intravenous or intra-arterial thrombolytic agents.[71]

Finally, the postprocedural use of antithrombotic agents continues to evolve, as we explore more complex options and push the boundaries of previous practices. For example, patients treated with IV-tPA are not supposed to receive any antithrombotic agents for the first 24 hours following treatment. However, this *dictum* conflicts with the needs of those who require urgent stenting during their rescue procedure since antithrombotic agents are necessary to prevent acute stent thrombosis. The trend at the present time is to use parenteral agents, with a shift to using shorter acting drugs (eg, cangrelor), allowing a more flexible approach to dosing, pausing, and transitioning to long-term oral agents.[72]

SUMMARY

Throughout the first quarter of the present century, neuroendovascular rescue has evolved considerably, and continues to do so. Starting with the simple intra-arterial instillation of thrombolytic agents via microcatheters to dissolve occluding thromboembolic material, the current status is one that includes a variety of different techniques such as direct aspiration of thrombus, thrombus removal by stent retriever, adjuvant techniques such as balloon angioplasty, stenting, and tactical intra-arterial instillation of thrombolytic agents in smaller branches to treat no reflow phenomenon. The trends continue to be the introduction of new devices and strategies with the objective of shortening the recanalization window as much as possible.

In parallel, the periprocedural care of these patients must be carefully orchestrated, as it provides a major framework that maximizes success in outcomes. Such care incorporates proper qualification of AIS patients for treatment allocation, hemodynamic management before, during and after the procedure is completed, incorporation of a follow-up antithrombotic regimens tailored to each clinical scenario, and overall clinical support.

CLINICS CARE POINTS

- Acute ischemic stroke caused by large arterial occlusion constitutes a well established indication for neuroendovascular rescue, irrespective of prior treatment with intravenous thrombolysis.

- Although patients with type I cerebral perfusion maps (ie, small ischemic core and large penumbra mismatch) demonstrate the ideal profile for benefiting from neuroendovascular rescue, those with larger ischemic core should also be considered for intervention.
- Although patients with large arterial occlusion presenting early (ie, a few hours) following onset are more likely to benefit from urgent intervention, those whose cerebral perfusion imaging is consistent with an optimal profile are also likely to benefit, even if late within the first 24 hours interval from onset.
- Optimal periprocedural management of intravascular management and blood pressure is of paramount importance to the final outcome of patients undergoing neuroendovascular rescue, and must be tailored to the specific cerebral hemodynamic status at every stage of care.

FUNDING

No funding to acknowledge.

REFERENCES

1. Campbell BCV, Donnan GA, Lees KR, et al. Endovascular stent thrombectomy: the new standard of care for large vessel ischaemic stroke. Lancet Neurol 2015;14(8):846–54.
2. Gomez CR, Wadlington VR, Terry JB, et al. Neuroendovascular rescue. Non-thrombolytic approach to acute brain ischemia. Crit Care Clin 1999;15(4):755–76.
3. Pressman E, Goldman H, Wang C, et al. A meta-analysis and systematic review of endovascular thrombectomy versus medical management for acute basilar artery occlusion. Clin Neurol Neurosurg 2023;234:107986.
4. Hao JH, Liu WD, Wang ZD, et al. [Retrospective analysis of mechanical thrombectomy for distal branch occlusion of middle cerebral artery]. Zhonghua Yixue Zazhi 2020;100(16):1240–4.
5. Salahuddin H, Espinosa A, Buehler M, et al. Mechanical Thrombectomy for Middle Cerebral Artery Division Occlusions: A Systematic Review and Meta-Analysis. Interv Neurol 2017;6(3–4):242–53.
6. Shi ZS, Loh Y, Walker G, et al. Clinical outcomes in middle cerebral artery trunk occlusions versus secondary division occlusions after mechanical thrombectomy: pooled analysis of the Mechanical Embolus Removal in Cerebral Ischemia (MERCI) and Multi MERCI trials. Stroke 2010;41(5):953–60.
7. Sallustio F, Pracucci G, Cappellari M, et al. Carotid artery stenting during endovascular thrombectomy for acute ischemic stroke with tandem occlusion: the Italian Registry of Endovascular Treatment in Acute Stroke. Acta Neurol Belg 2023; 123(2):475–85.
8. Farooqui M, Zaidat OO, Hassan AE, et al. Functional and safety outcomes of carotid artery stenting and mechanical thrombectomy for large vessel occlusion ischemic stroke with tandem lesions. JAMA Netw Open 2023;6(3):e230736.
9. Diana F, Romoli M, Toccaceli G, et al. Emergent carotid stenting versus no stenting for acute ischemic stroke due to tandem occlusion: a meta-analysis. J Neurointerventional Surg 2023;15(5):428–32.
10. Mohammaden MH, Tarek MA, Aboul Nour H, et al. Rescue intracranial stenting for failed posterior circulation thrombectomy: analysis from the Stenting and Angioplasty in NeuroThrombectomy (SAINT) study. J Neurointerventional Surg 2023. https://doi.org/10.1136/jnis-2023-020676.

11. Ifergan H, Dargazanli C, Ben Hassen W, et al. Rescue intracranial permanent stenting for refractory occlusion following thrombectomy: a propensity matched analysis. J Neurointerventional Surg 2023;16(2):115–23.

12. Cai J, Xu H, Xiao R, et al. Rescue intracranial stenting for acute ischemic stroke after the failure of mechanical thrombectomy: A systematic review, meta-analysis, and trial sequential analysis. Front Neurol 2023;14:1023089.

13. Abuelazm M, Ahmad U, Abu Suilik H, et al. Endovascular Thrombectomy for Acute Stroke with a Large Ischemic Core: A Systematic Review and Meta-Analysis of Randomized Controlled Trials. Clin Neuroradiol 2023;33(3):625–34.

14. Gory B, Finitsis S, Desilles JP, et al. Successful Thrombectomy Improves Functional Outcome in Tandem Occlusions with a Large Ischemic Core. World Neurosurg 2023;178:e282–91.

15. Kobeissi H, Adusumilli G, Ghozy S, et al. Endovascular thrombectomy for ischemic stroke with large core volume: An updated, post-TESLA systematic review and meta-analysis of the randomized trials. Intervent Neuroradiol 2023. 15910199231185738.

16. Wang J, Qiu J, Wang Y. Neurological functional independence after endovascular thrombectomy and different imaging modalities for large infarct core assessment : a systematic review and meta-analysis. Clin Neuroradiol 2023;33(1):21–9.

17. Burnette WC, Nesbit GM, Barnwell SL. Intra-arterial thrombolysis for acute stroke. Neuroimaging Clin N Am 1999;9(3):491–508.

18. Abou-Chebl A, Furlan AJ. Intra-arterial thrombolysis in acute stroke. Curr Opin Neurol 2000;13(1):51–5.

19. del Zoppo GJ, Higashida RT, Furlan AJ, et al. PROACT: a phase II randomized trial of recombinant pro-urokinase by direct arterial delivery in acute middle cerebral artery stroke. PROACT Investigators. Prolyse in Acute Cerebral Thromboembolism. Stroke 1998;29(1):4–11.

20. Furlan A, Higashida R, Wechsler L, et al. Intra-arterial prourokinase for acute ischemic stroke. The PROACT II study: a randomized controlled trial. Prolyse in Acute Cerebral Thromboembolism. JAMA 1999;282(21):2003–11.

21. Kerber CW, Barr JD, Berger RM, et al. Snare retrieval of intracranial thrombus in patients with acute stroke. J Vasc Intervent Radiol 2002;13(12):1269–74.

22. Schumacher HC, Meyers PM, Yavagal DR, et al. Endovascular mechanical thrombectomy of an occluded superior division branch of the left MCA for acute cardioembolic stroke. Cardiovasc Intervent Radiol 2003;26(3):305–8.

23. Gonzalez A, Mayol A, Martínez E, et al. Mechanical thrombectomy with snare in patients with acute ischemic stroke. Neuroradiology 2007;49(4):365–72.

24. Martinez H, Zoarski GH, Obuchowski AM, et al. Mechanical thrombectomy of the internal carotid artery and middle cerebral arteries for acute stroke by using the retriever device. AJNR Am J Neuroradiol 2004;25(10):1812–5.

25. Katz JM, Gobin YP. Merci Retriever in acute stroke treatment. Expet Rev Med Dev 2006;3(3):273–80.

26. Smith WS. Safety of mechanical thrombectomy and intravenous tissue plasminogen activator in acute ischemic stroke. Results of the multi Mechanical Embolus Removal in Cerebral Ischemia (MERCI) trial, part I. AJNR Am J Neuroradiol 2006; 27(6):1177–82.

27. Smith WS, Sung G, Saver J, et al. Mechanical thrombectomy for acute ischemic stroke: final results of the Multi MERCI trial. Stroke 2008;39(4):1205–12.

28. Costalat V, Machi P, Lobotesis K, et al. Rescue, combined, and stand-alone thrombectomy in the management of large vessel occlusion stroke using the

solitaire device: a prospective 50-patient single-center study: timing, safety, and efficacy. Stroke 2011;42(7):1929–35.

29. Nezzo M, et al. Aspiration thrombectomy of M2 segment in acute ischemic stroke: The clinical reality in a neurovascular reference center. Cardiovasc Revascularization Med 2023;55–9.

30. Molinaro S, Russo R, Mistretta F, et al. Maximizing the available space : the new RED 062 aspiration catheter in conjunction with 7F guide catheter in mechanical thrombectomy for left anterior circulation stroke via direct transradial approach. Clin Neuroradiol 2023;33(3):865–8.

31. Leone G, Muto M, Giordano F, et al. Initial experience using the new pHLO 0.072-inch Large-bore catheter for direct aspiration thrombectomy in acute ischemic stroke. Neurointervention 2023;18(1):30–7.

32. Xing PF, Yang PF, Li ZF, et al. Comparison of aspiration versus stent retriever thrombectomy as the preferred strategy for patients with acute terminal internal carotid artery occlusion: a propensity score matching analysis. AJNR Am J Neuroradiol 2020;41(3):469–76.

33. Almekhlafi MA, Goyal M, Dippel DWJ, et al. Healthy life-year costs of treatment speed from arrival to endovascular thrombectomy in patients with ischemic stroke: a meta-analysis of individual patient data from 7 randomized clinical trials. JAMA Neurol 2021;78(6):709–17.

34. Senturk C. Mechanical thrombectomy with a novel beveled tip aspiration catheter: A technical case report. Brain Circ 2022;8(4):215–8.

35. Vargas J, Blalock J, Venkatraman A, et al. Efficacy of beveled tip aspiration catheter in mechanical thrombectomy for acute ischemic stroke. J Neurointerventional Surg 2021;13(9):823–6.

36. Nogueira RG, Frei D, Kirmani JF, et al. Safety and efficacy of a 3-dimensional stent retriever with aspiration-based thrombectomy vs aspiration-based thrombectomy alone in acute ischemic stroke intervention: a randomized clinical trial. JAMA Neurol 2018;75(3):304–11.

37. Steglich-Arnholm H, Kondziella D, Wagner A, et al. Mechanical thrombectomy with the embolus retriever with interlinked cages in acute ischemic stroke: ERIC, the new boy in the class. AJNR Am J Neuroradiol 2017;38(7):1356–61.

38. Prothmann S, Lockau H, Dorn F, et al. The phenox clot retriever as part of a multimodal mechanical thrombectomy approach in acute ischemic stroke: single center experience in 56 patients. Sci World J 2012;2012:190763.

39. Will L, Maus V, Maurer C, et al. Mechanical thrombectomy in acute ischemic stroke using a manually expandable stent retriever (tigertriever) : preliminary single center experience. Clin Neuroradiol 2021;31(2):491–7.

40. Gruber P, Diepers M, von Hessling A, et al. Mechanical thrombectomy using the new Tigertriever in acute ischemic stroke patients - A Swiss prospective multicenter study. Intervent Neuroradiol 2020;26(5):598–601.

41. Kitazawa K, Ito Y, Koyama M, et al. Thrombectomy for small-artery occlusions with the small-diameter stent retriever, tron Fx 2 mm x 15 mm: a case series. J Neuroendovasc Ther 2021;15(5):332–8.

42. de Castro Afonso LH, Borghini Pazuello G, Seizem Nakiri G, et al. Thrombectomy for M2 occlusions and the role of the dominant branch. Intervent Neuroradiol 2019;25(6):697–704.

43. Gomez CR. Time is brain: the stroke theory of relativity. J Stroke Cerebrovasc Dis 2018;27(8):2214–27.

44. Gomez CR FB, Siddiq F, Qureshi AI. Triage of stroke patients for urgent intervention. In: Edgell RC CK, editor. Neurointervention in the medical specialties. A comprehensive guide. Switzerland: Humana Press; 2022. p. 73–91.

45. Nguyen TN, Abdalkader M, Nagel S, et al. Noncontrast computed tomography vs computed tomography perfusion or magnetic resonance imaging selection in late presentation of stroke with large-vessel occlusion. JAMA Neurol 2022; 79(1):22–31.

46. Karamchandani RR, Satyanarayana S, Yang H, et al. Predicting severe disability or death in endovascular thrombectomy with large computed tomography perfusion core infarction and limited penumbra. Intervent Neuroradiol 2023. 15910199231193466.

47. Koneru M, Hoseinyazdi M, Lakhani DA, et al. Redefining CT perfusion-based ischemic core estimates for the ghost core in early time window stroke. J Neuroimaging 2023;34(2):249–56.

48. Martins N, Aires A, Mendez B, et al. Ghost infarct core and admission computed tomography perfusion: redefining the role of neuroimaging in acute ischemic stroke. Interv Neurol 2018;7(6):513–21.

49. Rodrigues GM, Mohammaden MH, Haussen DC, et al. Ghost infarct core following endovascular reperfusion: A risk for computed tomography perfusion misguided selection in stroke. Int J Stroke 2021. 17474930211056228.

50. Xu XQ, Ma G, Lu SS, et al. Predictors of ghost infarct core on baseline computed tomography perfusion in stroke patients with successful recanalization after mechanical thrombectomy. Eur Radiol 2023;33(3):1792–800.

51. Kim BM, Baek JH, Heo JH, et al. Collateral status affects the onset-to-reperfusion time window for good outcome. J Neurol Neurosurg Psychiatry 2018;89(9):903–9.

52. Wijayatilake DS, Ratnayake G, Ragavan D. Anaesthesia for neuroradiology: thrombectomy: 'one small step for man, one giant leap for anaesthesia'. Curr Opin Anaesthesiol 2016;29(5):568–75.

53. Gomez CR, Cardonell B, Pfeiffer K, et al. Optimizing workflow of urgent stroke endovascular intervention: A focused lean six sigma project. J Stroke Cerebrovasc Dis 2024;33(3):107559.

54. Messer MP, Schönenberger S, Möhlenbruch MA, et al. Minor stroke syndromes in large-vessel occlusions: mechanical thrombectomy or thrombolysis only? AJNR Am J Neuroradiol 2017;38(6):1177–9.

55. Alexandre AM, Valente I, Frisullo G, et al. Mechanical thrombectomy in patients with stroke due to large vessel occlusion in the anterior circulation and low baseline NIHSS score. J Integr Neurosci 2021;20(3):645–50.

56. Alexandre AM, Valente I, Pedicelli A, et al. Mechanical thrombectomy in acute ischemic stroke due to large vessel occlusion in the anterior circulation and low baseline National Institute of Health Stroke Scale score: a multicenter retrospective matched analysis. Neurol Sci 2022;43(5):3105–12.

57. Yamazaki N, Kimura N, Doijiri R, et al. A low score on the National Institutes of Health Stroke Scale with eye movement disorder may indicate a good candidate for acute mechanical thrombectomy for posterior circulation large vessel occlusion: illustrative cases. J Neurosurg Case Lessons 2022;4(5).

58. Adams HP Jr, Brott TG, Furlan AJ, et al. Guidelines for thrombolytic therapy for acute stroke: a supplement to the guidelines for the management of patients with acute ischemic stroke. A statement for healthcare professionals from a Special Writing Group of the Stroke Council, American Heart Association. Circulation 1996;94(5):1167–74.

59. Ishfaq MF, Gulraiz S, Huang W, et al. Endovascular thrombectomy with or without intravenous thrombolysis: a meta-analysis of randomized controlled trials. Intervent Neuroradiol 2023;29(2):157–64.

60. Qureshi AI, Baskett WI, Bains NK, et al. Outcomes with IV tenecteplase and IV alteplase for acute ischemic stroke with or without thrombectomy in real-world settings in the United States. J Stroke Cerebrovasc Dis 2023;32(2):106898.

61. Powers WJ, Rabinstein AA, Ackerson T, et al. Guidelines for the early management of patients with acute ischemic stroke: 2019 update to the 2018 guidelines for the early management of acute ischemic stroke: a guideline for healthcare Professionals From the American Heart Association/American Stroke Association. Stroke 2019;50(12):e344–418.

62. Bellon RJ, Putman CM, Budzik RF, et al. Rheolytic thrombectomy of the occluded internal carotid artery in the setting of acute ischemic stroke. AJNR Am J Neuroradiol 2001;22(3):526–30.

63. Bulwa Z, Gomez CR, Morales-Vidal S, et al. Management of blood pressure after acute ischemic stroke. Curr Neurol Neurosci Rep 2019;19(29):1–13.

64. Kim BJ, Chung JW, Park HK, et al. CT angiography of collateral vessels and outcomes in endovascular-treated acute ischemic stroke patients. J Clin Neurol 2017;13(2):121–8.

65. Archer DP, Walker AM, McCann SK, et al. Anesthetic neuroprotection in experimental stroke in rodents: a systematic review and meta-analysis. Anesthesiology 2017;126(4):653–65.

66. Theron J, Nelson M, Alachkar F, et al. Dynamic digitized cerebral parenchymography. Neuroradiology 1992;34(4):361–4.

67. Nakagawa I, Kotsugi M, Yokoyama S, et al. Parenchymal Blood Volume Changes Immediately After Endovascular Thrombectomy Predict Futile Recanalization in Patients with Emergent Large Vessel Occlusion. World Neurosurg 2023;176: e711–8.

68. Zhang Y, Jiang M, Gao Y, et al. No-reflow" phenomenon in acute ischemic stroke. J Cerebr Blood Flow Metabol 2024;44(1):19–37.

69. Mujanovic A, Ng F, Meinel TR, et al. No-reflow phenomenon in stroke patients: A systematic literature review and meta-analysis of clinical data. Int J Stroke 2024; 19(1):58–67.

70. Jia M, Jin F, Li S, et al. No-reflow after stroke reperfusion therapy: An emerging phenomenon to be explored. CNS Neurosci Ther 2024;30(2):e14631.

71. Ebaid NY, Mouffokes A, Yasen NS, et al. Diagnostic accuracy of dual-energy computed tomography in the diagnosis of neurological complications after endovascular treatment of acute ischaemic stroke: a systematic review and meta-analysis. Br J Radiol 2024;97(1153):73–92.

72. Marnat G, Finistis S, Delvoye F, et al. Safety and efficacy of cangrelor in acute stroke treated with mechanical thrombectomy: endovascular treatment of ischemic stroke registry and meta-analysis. AJNR Am J Neuroradiol 2022; 43(3):410–5.

The Role of the Vascular Neurologist in Optimizing Stroke Care

Hannah J. Roeder, MD, MPH[a], Enrique C. Leira, MD, MS[a,b,c],*

KEYWORDS

- Vascular neurology • Fellowship training • Acute stroke care • Thrombolysis
- Endovascular thrombectomy • Stroke disparities

KEY POINTS

- Significant advances in stroke treatment have been made, which have transformed the role of the vascular neurologist.
- Expanded indications for reperfusion therapies have the potential to significantly benefit patients and improve public health but require universal immediate access to the expertise of vascular neurologists and imaging capabilities to optimize outcomes and minimize disparities.
- While the number of vascular neurology trainees and accredited subspecialists is growing, the field must make efforts to recruit a large and diverse group of trainees to adequately meet the expanding clinical demand.

INTRODUCTION/HISTORY/DEFINITIONS/BACKGROUND

Stroke is the leading cause of disability and the fifth leading cause of death in the United States. Approximately 800,000 people suffer a new or recurrent stroke each year in the United States.[1] Scientific knowledge and clinical care in acute stroke have progressed significantly in recent years. An expanding number of treatment opportunities require enough physicians with specialized training in cerebrovascular disorders to deliver up-to-date evidence-based care. Vascular neurologists play a key role in stroke systems of care across the spectrum from community education, acute stroke treatment, secondary prevention, and rehabilitation. The public health implications of an optimized stroke system of care are profound.

[a] Department of Neurology, University of Iowa Carver College of Medicine, 200 Hawkins Drive, Iowa City, IA, USA; [b] Department of Neurosurgery, University of Iowa Carver College of Medicine, 200 Hawkins Drive, Iowa City, IA, USA; [c] Department of Epidemiology, University of Iowa Carver College of Medicine, 200 Hawkins Drive, Iowa City, IA, USA
* Corresponding author. Department of Neurology, University of Iowa Carver College of Medicine, 200 Hawkins Drive, Iowa City, IA 52242.
E-mail address: enrique-leira@uiowa.edu

Neurol Clin 42 (2024) 739–752
https://doi.org/10.1016/j.ncl.2024.03.007
0733-8619/24/© 2024 Elsevier Inc. All rights reserved.

neurologic.theclinics.com

DISCUSSION
Vascular Neurology Training

Vascular neurologists, colloquially known as stroke doctors, are physicians who complete neurology or physical medicine residency training and have additional training and expertise in stroke and related cerebrovascular conditions. In recognition of the need *to officially establish the field of vascular neurology as a definite area of subspecialization in neurology and child neurology and to provide a means of identifying properly trained and experienced vascular neurologists*, the American Board of Psychiatry and Neurology (ABPN) began offering subspecialty certification in vascular neurology beginning in 2005.[2] From 2005 to 2009, the Practice Pathway Period, the ABPN granted certification to physicians who demonstrated sufficient experience in stroke neurology regardless of fellowship training ("legacied in"). Since 2012, the vascular neurology examination has been offered in even years only. Physicians with specialty certification in neurology or child neurology must now complete a 1 year Accreditation Council for Graduate Medical Education (ACGME)-accredited fellowship in vascular neurology prior to taking the biennial examination.[2] The number of certificates issued has steadily risen over the last few cycles of certification, since 2016, as illustrated in **Fig. 1**.[3] The rising number of newly certified vascular neurologists temporally corresponds with the publication of the first randomized clinical trials (RCTs) demonstrating efficacy of endovascular thrombectomy (EVT). While only speculative, the trend may reflect renewed excitement in the field of stroke among medical graduates.

As of the end of 2022, a total of 2264 certificates have been issued in the vascular neurology subspecialty. This total includes those issued to individuals who have since

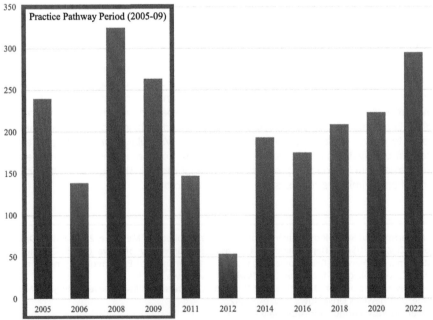

Fig. 1. Vascular neurology certifications issued by year. (*Data* from Neurology ABoPa. Certifications by Year—Subspecialties. https://www.abpn.org/wp-content/uploads/2023/03/Certifications-by-Year-Subspecialties-2022.pdf. 2023. Accessed 01 July 2023.)

switched fields, retired, or died. The ACGME estimates that approximately 1789 physicians with active certificates are practicing stroke neurologists.[4] As of the 2021 to 2022 academic year, there were 112 ACGME-approved vascular neurology fellowship programs in the United States, up from 92 programs in 2017 to 2018.[5] All programs combined to total 166 graduating vascular neurology fellows in 2022.[5]

Growing an adequate and diverse health care workforce is vital toward meeting the clinical demand while reducing disparities in neurology and stroke care. Reaching this goal starts with recruiting diverse trainees. While the growing number of fellowship programs and trainees in vascular neurology is beneficial toward meeting the growing demand for stroke care, data suggest a decline in trainees entering vascular neurology fellowship from racial and ethnic groups who have been historically marginalized and systemically excluded from medicine. One analysis found that the percentage of trainees from underrepresented racial and ethnic groups entering vascular neurology fellowship fell from 16.9% of all trainees in 2006 to 2009 to 9.3% in 2015 to 2018.[6] Similarly, women also remain underrepresented in vascular neurology fellowship programs.[7] According to ACGME data, only 39.7% of vascular neurology fellows in the 2021 to 2022 academic year self-identified as female; compared to 47.7% of adult neurology residents.[5] Demographically diverse physicians help ensure optimal health care delivery for patients across the sociodemographic spectrum. Key factors in choosing a medical fellowship may include subspecialty exposure during training, mentors and influential role models, work–life balance, educational debt and specialty compensation, and available research, education, and clinical opportunities.[7] Targeting these factors may help improve the diversity of physicians pursuing vascular neurology (**Fig. 2**).

Vascular Neurology Pathways

Vascular neurologists pursue a diverse range of additional training and professional positions. Some may have, or will pursue, additional training in neuroendovascular surgery, neurocritical care, and/or other neurologic subspecialties. They may also divide their time between clinical work and other professional pursuits, including research, quality improvement, education, administration, and public health.

Vascular neurologists with additional neurointerventional training often spend much of their clinical time performing endovascular procedures, including EVT to treat acute ischemic stroke and securing ruptured aneurysms, as well as other elective procedures to decrease the risk of stroke. The endovascular field has blossomed in recent years since the publication of RCTs of EVT, starting with MR CLEAN in 2015, demonstrating the efficacy of thrombectomy over medical management alone (including thrombolysis if indicated) in patients with a proximal large vessel occlusion (LVO).[8] Unlike vascular neurology, neuroendovascular surgery is a multi-specialty discipline and may be pursued after completing a residency in neurology, radiology, interventional radiology, or neurosurgery. As a relatively nascent subspecialty, the prerequisites, training pathways, and curricula are evolving. After residency, the neurologist pursuing neuroendovascular surgery must first complete a prerequisite fellowship in vascular neurology or neurocritical care prior to 2 years of neurointerventional training, consisting of a preliminary endovascular year and a neurointerventional treatment year.[9] The Committee for Advanced Subspecialty Training of the Society of Neurologic Surgeons provides accreditation to neuroendovascular surgery fellowships.[10] While the practice of vascular neurology and neurointerventional procedures can be balanced, disparate compensation for the two fields, higher for the latter, can be challenging for the provider and the health care organization.[11]

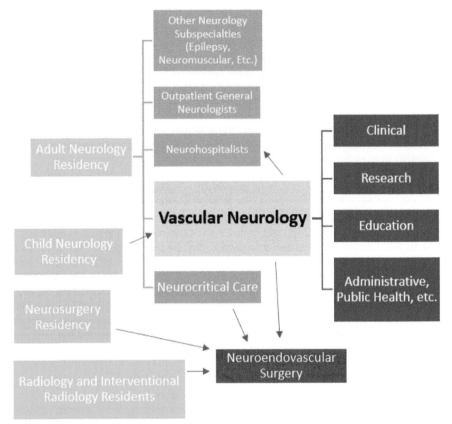

Fig. 2. Training and practice pathways for vascular neurologists.

Vascular neurologists with additional neurocritical care training may pursue a neuro-intensivist practice, instead or in addition to serving as a stroke physician. The ABPN recently started offering an examination toward certification in the neurocritical care subspecialty in 2021.[3] Other stroke-trained physicians may serve primarily in a neuro-hospitalist role, providing care for patients hospitalized with stroke and non-vascular neurologic conditions, from seizures to myasthenia to meningitis. Some vascular neurologists also choose to provide remote stroke care known as telestroke. Telestroke allows the expertise of vascular neurologists to be immediately available at more rural and remote locations that do not have a neurologist on-call and lead to prompt diagnoses and treatment recommendations, in addition to guiding secondary prevention. While telestroke helps mitigate the existing geographic disparity in vascular neurologists that plagues rural areas, it does not solve the overall shortage of specialists.

In addition to clinical responsibilities, a vascular neurologist's role may include other nonclinical professional activities, which may reduce their clinical full-time equivalents (cFTE). Stroke physicians may engage in all aspects of stroke translational research, from discovery to population health. Stroke research may include leading or participating in clinical trials of acute stroke treatments, secondary stroke prevention, or stroke recovery. Researchers may engage in epidemiologic studies, and others may use animal models of stroke. Vascular neurologists may also lead local quality improvement initiatives.

Education is an important aspect of improving cerebrovascular outcomes. Vascular neurologists may act as educators for multiple levels of trainees from undergraduates to fellows, as well as teaching colleagues in other health care disciplines and the community at large. Educational activities may include formal lecturing, clinical supervision, facilitating stroke simulations, mentoring, and fulfilling medical school and ACGME leadership roles. Given their comprehensive understanding of stroke care, vascular neurologists are also well suited for administrative leadership roles in both primary and comprehensive stroke centers. Stroke physicians may also be leaders in community health through managing stroke registries and leading public health campaigns.

Clinical Role of the Vascular Neurologist

Vascular neurology is a broad clinical discipline that spans emergency department acute consultations and interventions, inpatient care in intensive care and stroke units, and outpatient (clinic) settings. Vascular neurologists provide comprehensive expertise in the treatment, prevention, and rehabilitation of stroke, alongside an interdisciplinary team.

Vascular neurologists are leaders and a critical part of the multidisciplinary team that responds to code stroke activations.[12] The purpose of the code stroke is to decrease intrahospital delays in stroke care by providing rapid neurologic assessment and stabilization, while expediting safe and rapid acute stroke treatments for eligible patients. As in all medical emergencies, the team initially assesses circulation, airway, and breathing. In the case of stroke, such stabilization primarily focuses on blood pressure management to avoid harm from hypoperfusion in the ischemic penumbra, as well as assessing the ability to protect the airway from challenges such as decreased level of consciousness or dysphagia. The code stroke team also ensures adequate intravenous access, checks vital signs, obtains the appropriate laboratory tests, obtains a brief history, and performs a relevant neurologic examination, typically following the National Institutes of Health Stroke Scale format given its simplicity and prognostic value.[13] Code stroke patients typically require emergent neuroimaging; depending on the institution, this may include computed tomography or MR modalities. The expertise of the vascular neurologist includes performing the neurologic examination and interpreting the history, examination, neuroimaging, and other clinical data in the patient's overall clinical context in an expeditious manner. During a code stroke, the team led by vascular neurologists rapidly generates a differential diagnosis, identifies a stroke, makes recommendations regarding advanced imaging, counsels patients and families, administers thrombolytics when indicated, consults neuroendovascular surgery for thrombectomy-eligible patients, and triages patients to the appropriate level of care, while collaborating with nurses, pharmacists, other physicians, and other medical professionals to deliver care.

As code strokes were developed to avoid missing patients who may be eligible for timely therapies, activation criteria tend to be simple and sensitive rather than specific. As such, code strokes are often activated for patients who end up being diagnosed with neurologic deficits due to nonvascular causes, which are called stroke mimics. The incidence of mimics among code stroke activations is estimated to be about 20% but varies considerably between studies based on clinical setting, patient demographics, institutional protocols, and diagnostic practices and exceeds 50% in some settings.[14,15] Seizure, migraine, and other headache syndromes, syncope, functional neurologic disorder, vestibular disorder, psychiatric disease, and toxic-metabolic infectious abnormalities are frequently encountered stroke mimics.[16] Vascular neurologists must be familiar with the presentation and initial management of common stroke mimics, which are also medical emergencies. As a result of institutional code stroke protocols, vascular neurologists are often the first neurologists to assess and provide recommendations for patients with a wide range of acute neurologic emergencies. While some rate of code stroke activation for mimics is inevitable to avoid missing patients eligible for acute stroke treatment, the management of stroke mimics nevertheless creates additional clinical workload and consult burden which can negatively impact the efficiency of the stroke service and contribute to burnout. A more efficient model would allow for the vascular neurologist to triage stroke mimics to the most appropriate service after diagnosis, stabilization, and initial treatment. MR imaging may help differentiate stroke from mimic but is usually not immediately available and is time-consuming. Stroke mimics may be treated with thrombolytics as a presumed ischemic stroke. Stroke mimics often require admission to inpatient stroke services for further diagnostic and therapeutic management.

In the setting of transient focal neurologic deficits, an accurate diagnosis relies even more on clinical history. Transient ischemic attacks (TIAs) are transient neurologic deficits due to ischemia of the brain, spinal cord, or retina, often of 5 to 10 minutes in duration, which does not result in infarction.[17] TIAs are frequently misdiagnosed, and a vascular neurology consult may help determine which patients could benefit from additional neurovascular evaluation and when stroke prophylactic treatments are indicated. In addition to arterial ischemic strokes (AISs), hemorrhagic strokes, and TIAs, vascular neurologists manage other conditions affecting the cerebrovascular system including cortical and cerebral sinus venous thrombosis, arteriopathies such as cervical and intracranial arterial atherosclerosis or dissection, vascular malformations, and other cerebral and spinal cord vascular abnormalities.

Patients requiring hospitalization for acute cerebrovascular disease benefit from treatment in an acute stroke unit, an organized inpatient setting dedicated to managing stroke patients and the common post-stroke complications.[18] A stroke unit ensures patients access to a multidisciplinary team, including specialized nursing, pharmacy, physical therapy, occupational therapy, speech and language pathologists, physicians, and other professionals, and is associated with lower mortality and greater independence following stroke.[18] On the inpatient unit, vascular neurologists guide the diagnostic work-up of stroke etiology, implement appropriate secondary stroke prevention, and work with therapists to establish an appropriate rehabilitation plan, during admission and on discharge.

Vascular neurologists also see patients with chronic stroke and other cerebrovascular conditions in the outpatient setting. One purpose of the stroke clinic visit includes ensuring that a thorough stroke work-up has been completed. In the case of cryptogenic stroke, the vascular neurologist follows up on studies that may have been pending on hospital discharge and determines what further etiologic evaluation is needed. Clinic visits also allow ongoing patient education on lifestyle modification (such as smoking cessation, physical activity, and diet) and stroke risk factors, signs, and symptoms. The stroke clinician can monitor for post-stroke complications, such as post-stroke depression or spasticity, and make appropriate recommendations and referrals as needed. In post-stroke follow-up, vascular neurologists also assess for medication adherence and adverse effects and make medication adjustments as indicated. Additionally, the outpatient visits provide an opportunity for patients to participate in available secondary prevention and recovery clinical trials.

Evolving Stroke Care

Scientific knowledge and clinical care in acute stroke progressed significantly in recent decades. The publication of the National Institute of Neurological Disorders and Stroke (NINDS) tissue-type plasminogen activator (tPA) Stroke Trials in 1995 marks what may be considered the modern era of stroke care.[19] The study demonstrated the effectiveness of thrombolytic therapy administered within 3 hours of symptom onset in improving functional outcomes at 90 days for patients with acute AIS. ECASS III demonstrated tPA efficacy up to 4.5 hours from last known well (LKW).[20] Gradual adoption of thrombolytic use for stroke patients across the United States led health care systems to institute "Code Stroke" systems to minimize door-to-needle times. Many stroke patients are not eligible for thrombolytics due to delayed presentation. More recent trials suggest that selected patients with AIS with unknown LKW or LKW beyond 4.5 hours may benefit from thrombolytic administration guided by advanced imaging (EXTEND and WAKE-UP).[21,22]

Despite thrombolytic administration, patients with severe strokes caused by a proximal LVO continued to have largely poor outcomes. Clinician researchers began to investigate the role of endovascular therapy in acute stroke treatment. After several negative RCTs (SYNTHESIS, MR RESCUE, IMS III),[23–25] in 2015, MR CLEAN marked the first positive RCT demonstrating improved outcomes in patients with LVO receiving endovascular thrombectomy (EVT) within 6 hours from symptom onset compared with medical management alone.[8] Additional RCTs confirmed the efficacy of EVT, and subsequent trials (DAWN, DEFUSE) expanded the time frame for EVT up to 24 hours for patients with LVO and small established infarct (core) volumes.[26,27] Most recently RCTs published in early 2023, which are not yet reflected in clinical guidelines, demonstrated efficacy of treating patients who present with anterior circulation LVO with EVT up to 24 hours from LKW even with a larger core infarct present.[28,29]

In less time than a typical physician career span, stroke care underwent a seismic shift from therapeutic nihilism to a "time-is-brain" mantra with multiple medical and endovascular options available. To capitalize on transforming scientific breakthroughs into improved patient outcomes, the health care system must prioritize the provision of acute stroke care. The American Stroke Association publishes recommendations for establishment of stroke systems of care to guide best practices for translating scientific advances and clinical care innovations into improvements in patient outcomes.[30] Vascular neurologists are at the heart of such improvements.

Challenges and Opportunities for Vascular Neurologists

While vascular neurology is an exciting, dynamic specialty with substantial recent advances, the field continues to face challenges, including (1) supply issues, (2) growing demand, and (3) disparities in care (**Table 1**).

Supply challenges

The supply–demand imbalance in the acute stroke work force was identified in a paper a decade ago, which outlined concerns regarding whether the number of vascular neurologists trained each year was sufficient to meet the growing clinical demand.[31] The paper, published prior to the successful endovascular trials, argued that the oversupply of neurointerventionalists contributed to the shortage of vascular neurologists. Contemporary papers even proposed such draconian solutions as the indefinite suspension of neurointerventional fellowships.[32] Both the fields of vascular neurology and neuroendovascular surgery have greatly changed in the decade since those papers, particularly with the explosion of positive neuroendovascular trials; however, concerns regarding the shunting to neurointerventional practice remain relevant today. The establishment of thrombectomy as a standard therapy may further contribute to the shunting of vascular neurologists to a better remunerated endovascular career.

Table 1
Challenges, contributors, and potential solutions in the field of vascular neurology

Challenge	Contributors	Potential Solutions
Supply and Demand	• Supply: Shunting vascular neurologists to neurointerventional and other subspecialties • Demand: Aging population, obesity and diabetes epidemic, increasing stroke in the young • More emergent decision-making: Expanded indications for reperfusion therapies and greater use of advanced imaging	• More training opportunities and incentives to attract and retain vascular neurologists (eg, comparable remuneration, better work–life balance) • Vascular neurology extenders in stroke care (eg, advanced practice providers) • Employing technological advancements (eg, telestroke, artificial intelligence for neuroimaging)
Disparities in Stroke Outcomes	• Unequal geographic distribution of human and structural resources to treat stroke. • Racial, ethnic, and gender inequities in stroke care and outcomes.	• Use of maximal coverage models to locate stroke treatment resources while designing stroke systems of care • Expand telestroke, remote stroke resources, and stroke interventions during emergent transportation. • Recruit a more diverse vascular neurology workforce (diverse mentor networks, improved compensation packages, student loan forgiveness, and equal opportunities)

According to the American Academy of Neurology, the median compensation for a stroke physician is less than half that of a neurointerventionalist.[11] Additionally, in the thrombectomy era of stroke care, many perceive a glorification of endovascular care over medical interventions. Vascular neurologists responding to stroke codes may be seen as having a lesser role in the management of LVO, acting as mere facilitators to the impactful neurointerventional procedures. The reality is that the role for endovascular treatment in stroke has greatly expanded but so too has the medical care for patients with stroke. In fact, most patients with stroke only require medical care and do not have an indication for intervention.[33] The expertise and medical management provided by vascular neurologists remains essential, not only for maximizing stroke outcomes in those patients who undergo neurointervention, but for the greater number of those who do not need one.

Promisingly, a growing number of physicians are receiving vascular neurology training. In the last decade, the estimated number of practicing ACGME-certified vascular neurologists in the United States has increased from 1115 to 1789 (~38% increase).[4,31] Meanwhile, the stroke incidence in the United States has remained relatively steady, around 800,000 per year over this time.[1] As a result, from 2012 to 2022, the estimated number of strokes per certified vascular neurologist per year has decreased from 717 to 447. The ideal ratio of strokes per vascular neurologist is unknown. Additionally, this number is a limited reflection of the supply and demand as it does not account for vascular neurology-trained physicians who are shunted to other subspecialties and spend part or all their time performing neurohospitalist, neurointerventionalist, neurocritical, or other related clinical work. The figure also does not include other conditions which vascular neurologists manage (including TIAs, stroke mimics, and other cerebrovascular conditions) nor factor in nonclinical (research, education, etc.) time. Conversely, the calculation does not reflect that some stroke patients do not receive care from a vascular neurologist. Nevertheless, growth in the field is welcomed as the demand for vascular neurology expertise expands. The vascular neurology field urgently needs planning and resources to adjust its supply to the current and future demands.

Demand challenges

The demand for vascular neurology expertise is increasing due to multiple factors. While the incidence of stroke has stayed relatively level in recent years, demographic and socioeconomic factors threaten to spur increased stroke incidence in coming years. Declining deaths due to vascular disease, including strokes, was cited by the Centers for Disease Control and Prevention (CDC) as 1 of the 10 great public health achievements of the twentieth century.[34] The CDC attributed the achievement to declining tobacco use and improved detection and treatment of stroke risk factors, such as hypertension. In recent years, stroke incidence has stabilized but has increased in the young.[35] An aging population coupled with the ongoing obesity and diabetes epidemic in the United States suggest stroke incidence may grow and the demand for stroke care will thus increase, as well.

The scientific breakthroughs described have led to an exponential increase in treatment decisions that require more nuanced decision-making and advanced knowledge of cerebrovascular diseases. Recent RCT findings allow more patients to be eligible for reperfusion therapies. The successful implementation of updated best practice requires greater consultation with vascular neurologists. Extended-time windows for reperfusion lead to more stroke code activations and hence a greater demand for vascular neurologists to provide cognitive expertise in emergent situations. The delineation of which patients are eligible for reperfusion therapies using advanced imaging, such as perfusion studies and MR imaging, requires additional resources and time for imaging acquisition, as well as the expertise of the stroke neurologist to review the imaging and interpret the findings within the patient's clinical context. Growing use of reperfusion therapies requires greater utilization of intensive care units for post-stroke monitoring, which requires additional critical care time from vascular neurologists. Through improved acute stroke care delivery, thankfully more patients are surviving hospitalization for stroke, which also leads to a greater volume of patients who need stroke doctors to optimize evaluation, secondary prevention, and other post-stroke management. As such, the demand for vascular neurology expertise will likely continue to grow.

Improving the supply and demand

Several strategies may be used simultaneously to improve the supply–demand challenge facing vascular neurology. The growing number of vascular neurology fellowships (and fellows) in recent years has led to the opportunity to train more vascular neurologists. Attracting physicians into vascular neurology and retaining them in the field (avoiding shunting into interventional training and practice, for example) will require making the field more attractive to physicians-in-training. Some measures may include fast-track training programs to reduce total years spent in residency and fellowship and programs addressing educational debt. Other possibilities are democratized reimbursement rates that financially equate cognitive stroke work to the same degree as interventional work. Another opportunity is to improve the stroke burden of vascular neurologists to have a better work–life balance with greater distribution of night, weekend, and holiday call.[36] In addition to attracting and retaining physicians in vascular neurology, the supply of health care providers caring for stroke patients may still be insufficient to meet the demand. Meeting the demand will require supplementation from advance practice providers, hospitalists, and general neurologists to adequately care for all patients with stroke. We envision vascular neurologists leading such multidisciplinary groups and providing cross-training to disseminate stroke cognitive expertise. Technological efforts may also improve the supply–demand imbalance. Telestroke is used to help vascular neurologists provide care for rural and remote patients in a timely manner. Artificial intelligence is already used in acute stroke neuroimaging interpretation and may be further employed to enhance providers that lack timely access to the required expertise.[37]

Improving the number and location of stroke centers

In 2003, the Joint Commission established a stroke center certification program.[38] Primary stroke centers have a 24/7 stroke team with a neurologist available either in person or via telemedicine, dedicated stroke beds, and the ability to administer thrombolytics. Thrombectomy-capable Centers must meet the Primary Stroke Center requirements and have intensive care beds dedicated to stroke patients and ability to perform EVT 24/7. The highest designation is the Comprehensive Stroke Center (CSC). At this level of care, hospitals, in addition to the requirements of the Thrombectomy-capable Center, must have 24/7 neurosurgical capabilities, meet the needs of multiple complex stroke patients, offer research, and meet increased education requirements for staff caring for stroke patients.[38] Understandably, most CSCs, which total between 150 and 200 hospitals in the United States, are located in large urban areas. In many locations, regional stroke care is provided via a hub-and-spoke model with the hub (CSC) providing consultation to other centers located in less populated rural areas. The location of stroke centers in the United States is determined, unfortunately, by market forces. Using maximal coverage models would result in a substantial better population coverage for the given resources.[39] Another challenge is the best triage option for patients in the field. The system must be tailored to the resources of a particular region. In heavily populated areas, mobile stroke units help extend the outreach of the CSC.[40] The goal is to minimize both door-to-needle and door-to-groin times for all patients.[33]

Stroke disparities and addressing inequities

While great strides in stroke care delivery have been made through scientific discovery and developing stroke care systems, those advances have not benefitted all patients equally. Access to stroke care and stroke outcomes are not uniform across the country, and vascular neurologists have a role in addressing such disparities. Stroke disparities, preventable differences in the burden of disease experienced by socially disadvantaged populations, are a significant public health problem. As CSCs are concentrated in urban areas and reperfusion therapies are time-dependent, geographic location is a significant barrier to stroke treatment. Rural patients with AIS are less likely to receive thrombolysis and less likely to undergo thrombectomy, they also have higher in-hospital mortality following stroke.[41] Telestroke and established referral protocols to allow rapid consultation with a vascular neurologist and streamlined transfer of patients who are potential thrombectomy candidates to capable centers may help improve outcomes for rural patients. Additionally, policy changes should address lengthy prehospital times owing to shortfalls in rural emergency medical services. Disparities in acute stroke treatment by race and ethnicity also exist in the United States. The reasons for the disparity are complex and include factors ranging from delayed recognition by patients or providers, mistrust of the health care system, or differential treatment. Addressing the root causes will require a multipronged approach.[42] Stroke physicians must advocate for policies at the hospital-level and beyond that promote equitable access for vulnerable communities. A diverse, well-trained vascular neurology work force will help mitigate such disparities. Reaching vulnerable populations often starts with training diverse clinicians. Efforts at multiple levels are needed to recruit a diverse workforce in vascular neurology, including diverse mentor networks, improved compensation packages and student loan forgiveness programs, and equal opportunities for research, grants, speakerships, promotion, and awards.

SUMMARY

Over the last 3 decades, the vascular neurology field has transitioned from contemplation and nihilism to a vibrant emergent field of effective therapies for acute strokes. Hospitals must now have 24/7 coverage by vascular neurologists, or alternatively the ability to rapidly consult with hospitals that have such coverage, to facilitate optimal selection of patients for acute stroke treatment. Vascular neurology is a dynamic subspecialty that has been transformed by the recent scientific advances and offers many potential clinical and professional avenues. However, the specialty faces significant challenges in providing a supply that adequately meets societal demands and organization of the stroke systems to optimize the provision of stroke care across geographic and demographic barriers. Meeting these challenges has the potential to greatly improve public cerebrovascular health.

CLINICS CARE POINTS

- Vascular neurology is an accredited, rewarding subspecialty with many potential professional and clinical opportunities.
- The demand for vascular neurology expertise continues to grow as universal access to readily available advanced knowledge of cerebrovascular diseases is needed to optimize delivery of acute stroke care.
- Multi-pronged efforts are required for the supply of vascular neurology expertise to meet the growing demand.
- Inequities in stroke care and outcomes persist across geography and demographics, and vascular neurologists have an important role in addressing stroke disparities.

DISCLOSURE

Dr. H.J. Roeder has no financial disclosures. Dr. E.C. Leira receives salary support from the NIH, United States-NINDS and is the vice chair of the Vascular Neurology Examination Writing Committee of the American Board of Psychiatry and Neurology.

REFERENCES

1. Tsao CW, Aday AW, Almarzooq ZI, et al, American Heart Association Council on Epidemiology and Prevention Statistics Committee and Stroke Statistics Subcommittee. Heart disease and stroke statistics—2023 update: a report from the American Heart Association. Circulation 2023;147:e93–621.
2. Neurology ABoPa. Vascular Neurology. 2023. Available at: https://abpn.org/become-certified/taking-a-subspecialty-exam/vascular-neurology/.

3. Neurology ABoPa. Certifications by Year—Subspecialties. 2023. Available at: https://www.abpn.org/wp-content/uploads/2023/03/Certifications-by-Year-Subspecialties-2022.pdf. [Accessed 1 July 2023].

4. Neurology ABoPa. Certifications —Total and Active. 2023. Available at: https://www.abpn.org/wp-content/uploads/2023/03/ABPN-Certifications-Total-and-Active-2022.pdf. [Accessed 1 July 2023].

5. Education ACfGM. Data resource book, academic year 2021-2022. Accreditation Council for Graduate Medical Education; 2022. Available at: https://www.acgme.org/globalassets/pfassets/publicationsbooks/2021-2022_acgme__databook_document.pdf. [Accessed 1 July 2023].

6. Das S, Farkas N, Binkley M, et al. Trends in racial and ethnic diversity in vascular neurology fellowships from 2006 to 2018: a cross-sectional analysis. Stroke 2022; 53:867–74.

7. Maqsood H, Naveed S, Younus S, et al. Gender and racial trends among vascular neurology fellowship programs: by design or by default. Cureus 2021;13.

8. Berkhemer OA, Fransen PS, Beumer D, et al, MR CLEAN Investigators. A randomized trial of intraarterial treatment for acute ischemic stroke. N Engl J Med 2015;372:11–20.

9. Surgery SoN. how to become a neurointerventionalist. 2023. Available at: https://www.snisonline.org/pathways/. [Accessed 1 July 2023].

10. Training CTCoAS. CNS endovascular surgery. 2023. Available at: https://sns-cast.org/cast-approved-fellowship-programs-in-cns-endovascular-surgery/. [Accessed 1 July 2023].

11. Neurology AAo. neurology compensation and productivity report. AAN 2021. Available at: https://www.aan.com/siteassets/home-page/tools-and-resources/practicing-neurologist–administrators/benchmarking-data/neurology-compensation–productivity/21_ncp_report.pdf. [Accessed 1 July 2023].

12. Gomez CR, Malkoff MD, Sauer CM, et al. Code stroke. An attempt to shorten in-hospital therapeutic delays. Stroke 1994;25:1920–3.

13. Adams H, Davis P, Leira E, et al. Baseline NIH Stroke Scale score strongly predicts outcome after stroke: a report of the Trial of Org 10172 in Acute Stroke Treatment (TOAST). Neurology 1999;53:126.

14. Nouh A, Amin-Hanjani S, Furie KL, et al. Identifying best practices to improve evaluation and management of in-hospital stroke: a scientific statement from the American Heart Association. Stroke 2022;53:e165–75.

15. McClelland G, Rodgers H, Flynn D, et al. The frequency, characteristics and aetiology of stroke mimic presentations: a narrative review. Eur J Emerg Med 2019; 26:2–8.

16. Pohl M, Hesszenberger D, Kapus K, et al. Ischemic stroke mimics: a comprehensive review. J Clin Neurosci 2021;93:174–82.

17. Sacco RL, Kasner SE, Broderick JP, et al, American Heart Association Stroke Council, Council on Cardiovascular Surgery and Anesthesia, Council on Cardiovascular Radiology and Intervention, Council on Cardiovascular and Stroke Nursing, Council on Epidemiology and Prevention, Council on Peripheral Vascular Disease, Council on Nutrition, Physical Activity and Metabolism. An updated definition of stroke for the 21st century: a statement for healthcare professionals from the American Heart Association/American Stroke Association. Stroke 2013;44:2064–89.

18. Langhorne P, Ramachandra S, Collaboration SUT. Organised inpatient (stroke unit) care for stroke: network meta-analysis. Cochrane Database Syst Rev 2020;4(4):CD000197.

19. Disorders NIoN, Group Sr-PSS. Tissue plasminogen activator for acute ischemic stroke. N Engl J Med 1995;333:1581–8.
20. Hacke W, Kaste M, Fieschi C, et al. Intravenous thrombolysis with recombinant tissue plasminogen activator for acute hemispheric stroke: the European Cooperative Acute Stroke Study (ECASS). JAMA 1995;274:1017–25.
21. Ma H, Campbell BC, Parsons MW, et al, EXTEND Investigators. Thrombolysis guided by perfusion imaging up to 9 hours after onset of stroke. N Engl J Med 2019;380:1795–803.
22. Thomalla G, Simonsen CZ, Boutitie F, et al, WAKE-UP Investigators. MRI-guided thrombolysis for stroke with unknown time of onset. N Engl J Med 2018;379:611–22.
23. Ciccone A, Valvassori L, Nichelatti M, et al, SYNTHESIS Expansion Investigators. Endovascular treatment for acute ischemic stroke. N Engl J Med 2013;368:904–13.
24. Kidwell CS, Jahan R, Gornbein J, et al, MR RESCUE Investigators. A trial of imaging selection and endovascular treatment for ischemic stroke. N Engl J Med 2013;368:914–23.
25. Broderick JP, Palesch YY, Demchuk AM, et al, Interventional Management of Stroke IMS III Investigators. Endovascular therapy after intravenous t-PA versus t-PA alone for stroke. N Engl J Med 2013;368:893–903.
26. Nogueira RG, Jadhav AP, Haussen DC, et al, DAWN Trial Investigators. Thrombectomy 6 to 24 hours after stroke with a mismatch between deficit and infarct. N Engl J Med 2018;378:11–21.
27. Albers GW, Marks MP, Kemp S, et al, DEFUSE 3 Investigators. Thrombectomy for stroke at 6 to 16 hours with selection by perfusion imaging. N Engl J Med 2018;378:708–18.
28. Sarraj A, Hassan AE, Abraham MG, et al, SELECT2 Investigators. Trial of endovascular thrombectomy for large ischemic strokes. N Engl J Med 2023;388:1259–71.
29. Huo X, Ma G, Tong X, et al, ANGEL-ASPECT Investigators. Trial of endovascular therapy for acute ischemic stroke with large infarct. N Engl J Med 2023;388:1272–83.
30. Adeoye O, Nyström KV, Yavagal DR, et al. Recommendations for the establishment of stroke systems of care: a 2019 update: a policy statement from the American Stroke Association. Stroke 2019;50:e187–210.
31. Leira EC, Kaskie B, Froehler MT, et al. The growing shortage of vascular neurologists in the era of health reform: planning is brain. Stroke 2013;44:822–7.
32. Fiorella D, Hirsch JA, Woo HH, et al. Should neurointerventional fellowship training be suspended indefinitely? J Neurointerv Surg 2012;4(5):315–8.
33. Leira EC, Savitz SI. In the era of thrombectomy, let us also protect the majority of patients with stroke who only require medical treatment. Stroke 2018;49:1538–40.
34. Control CfD. Prevention. Ten great public health achievements–United States, 1900-1999. MMWR Morbidity and Mortality Weekly Report 1999;48:241–3.
35. Boot E, Ekker MS, Putaala J, et al. Ischaemic stroke in young adults: a global perspective. J Neurol Neurosurg Psychiatr 2020;91:411–7.
36. Kenton EJ, Culebras A, Fayad PB, et al, AAN Vascular Neurology Stroke Practice Resources Workgroup. Impact of stroke call on the stroke neurology workforce in the United States: possible challenges and opportunities. J Stroke Cerebrovasc Dis 2018;27:2019–25.
37. Davenport T, Kalakota R. The potential for artificial intelligence in healthcare. Future Healthcare Journal 2019;6:94.

38. Commission TJ. Advanced Stroke Certifications. The Joint Commission. 2023. Available at: https://www.jointcommission.org/what-we-offer/certification/certifications-by-setting/hospital-certifications/stroke-certification/advanced-stroke/. [Accessed 1 July 2023].

39. Leira EC, Fairchild G, Segre AM, et al. Primary stroke centers should be located using maximal coverage models for optimal access. Stroke 2012;43:2417–22.

40. Ehntholt MS, Parasram M, Mir SA, et al. Mobile stroke units: bringing treatment to the patient. Curr Treat Options Neurol 2020;22:1–11.

41. Hammond G, Luke AA, Elson L, et al. Urban-rural inequities in acute stroke care and in-hospital mortality. Stroke 2020;51:2131–8.

42. Oh DM, Markovic D, Towfighi A. Race, Ethnic, Sex, and Socioeconomic Inequities in Interhospital Transfer for Acute Ischemic Stroke in the United States. Stroke 2023;54:1320–9.

Role of Stroke Scales and Scores in Cerebrovascular Disease

Violiza Inoa, MD[a,b,c],*,[1], Nitin Goyal, MD[a,b,c,2]

KEYWORDS

- Stroke scale • Stroke severity • Neurologic assessment • Outcome measures
- Stroke outcome

KEY POINTS

- Stroke scales are essential for planning treatment, predicting outcomes, and providing valuable support in guiding stroke patients through their recovery.
- An effective stroke scale should be reliable, comprehensive, user-friendly, widely validated, and demonstrate high sensitivity and specificity.
- As 1 scale will not cover all aspects of post-stroke disability, using a global outcome statistical model that integrates multiple scales is worth considering in future stroke trials.

INTRODUCTION

Stroke is a leading cause of disability and mortality worldwide. Despite primary and secondary stroke prevention measures, the global burden of stroke remains high. Over the past decade, the landscape of stroke treatment has undergone significant advancements. It evolved from intravenous thrombolysis being the only emergent intervention into endovascular treatment for acute strokes with large vessel occlusion (LVO).[1] Good outcomes with modern stroke treatments hinge on accurate and timely identification of the pathology. Pre-hospital care has emerged as an essential target for early identification of stroke patients who would benefit from rapid intervention. To that effect, various prehospital stroke scales were designed to guide the public and pre-hospital emergency personnel in triage.[2] However, such scales are not perfect, with variable sensitivities and specificities. Predictive value of some prehospital

[a] Semmes Murphey Clinic; [b] Department of Neurology, University of Tennessee Health Science Center, Memphis, TN, USA; [c] Department of Neurosurgery, University of Tennessee Health Science Center, Memphis, TN, USA
[1] Present address: 5868 Garden Oak Cove, Memphis, TN 38120.
[2] Present address: 5345 Shady Grove Road, Memphis, TN 38120.
* Corresponding author. 6325 Humphreys Boulevard, Memphis, TN 38120.
E-mail address: vinoa@semmes-murphey.com
Twitter: @InoaVioliza (V.I.)

Neurol Clin 42 (2024) 753–765
https://doi.org/10.1016/j.ncl.2024.03.008
0733-8619/24/© 2024 Elsevier Inc. All rights reserved.
neurologic.theclinics.com

stroke scales for the recognition of LVO remains low.[3] Various scales focus on identification of neurologic deficits, assessment of outcomes, and prediction of quality of life. However, no single scale has been able to capture the various sequelae of stroke on patients' lives. In this article, the authors provide an overview of commonly used stroke scales in emergency prehospital and hospital settings that are being used for the diagnosis, as well as the assessment of disability and quality of life of stroke patients.

DISCUSSION
Stroke Scales

Within this article, the authors have organized scales based on their applications in clinical practice. The authors' goal is to present a thorough overview of the commonly utilized scales, along with practical insights to facilitate a better understanding of their functions. Additionally, the authors discuss some of the limitations inherent to various scales. **Table 1** summarizes the most commonly used stroke scales in clinical practice and research.

Prehospital scales

Our current ability to treat stroke patients effectively largely depends on the early identification of stroke symptoms by the emergency medical service (EMS) personnel. As mechanical thrombectomy (MT) remains the standard of care for LVO stroke, the importance of identifying patients who may be eligible for MT has grown. There are potential advantages in bypassing primary stroke centers in favor of direct transportation to MT-capable centers. [4–6] Hence, the utilization of prehospital stroke scales has gained increasing significance in identifying patients who should be directly transported to advanced treatment facilities.

Prehospital stroke scales are developed as simplified versions of more comprehensive scales, such as the National Institutes of Health Stroke Scale (NIHSS), to serve as practical clinical assessments that can be employed by paramedics. Even in regions with well-established triage pathways for stroke care, EMS personnel perform suboptimally, missing over a third of stroke cases in the field.[7] Educational curriculums that include stroke protocols and assessments mimicking real-life scenarios have been proven to enhance EMS understanding of prehospital stroke severity scales and severity-based field triage protocols.[8] In addition, the documentation of a prehospital stroke scale is linked to improved EMS stroke recognition.[9]

Pitfalls

Prospective studies validating prehospital scales and comparing their performance are limited. Despite the likelihood that EMS education will help disseminate the use of prehospital stroke scales, there is a need for scientific evidence demonstrating that such education results in improved real-world performance. In addition, the clinical benefit associated with improved diagnostic accuracy of these scales has not been quantified. Among these, Rapid Arterial occlusion Evaluation (RACE) is the only scale that has undergone extensive field validation.[10,11] In the Netherlands, a study of 1039 people with suspected stroke found that prehospital scales detect anterior circulation LVO with acceptable-to-good accuracy. Participating paramedics assessed patients using a combination of 9 items from 8 prehospital stroke scales, including RACE, Los Angeles Motor Scale (LAMS), Cincinnati Stroke Triage Assessment Tool (C-STAT), Gaze-Face-Arm-Speech-Time (G-FAST), Prehospital Acute Stroke Severity (PASS), Conveniently-Grasped Field Assessment Stroke Triage (CG-FAST), Face-Arm-Speech-Time plus severe arm or leg deficit (FAST-PLUS), and Cincinnati Prehospital Stroke Scale

Table 1
Commonly used stroke scales

Stroke Scales	Items Tested	Background	Characteristics
Pre-Hospital Stroke Scales			
Face Arm Speech Test (FAST)	Face, arm, speech Other versions of the scale include balance, gaze, eye symptoms, and neglect	Developed in 1998 for EMS education in the United Kingdom	Initial studies showed PPV 64%–77% Multiple alternative versions have been created to increased sensitivity and specificity: BE-FAST, NEWFAST, FAST PLUS, FAST-ED, Gaze-Face-Arm-Speech-Time (G-FAST)
Cincinnati Prehospital Stroke Scale (CPSS)	Face, arm, speech	First validated in 1998 as a 3-item scale based on a simplification of the National Institutes of Health Stroke Scale (NIHSS), by the University of Cincinnati in Ohio, United States	Reported high sensitivity: 79%–94% for identification of patients with anterior circulation strokes
Los Angeles Prehospital Stroke Screen (LAPSS)	Face, handgrip, arm strength Four history items Blood glucose	Its prospective validation was published in 2000. It was developed as a stroke recognition tool designed specifically for prehospital personnel by the University of California at Los Angeles (UCLA) Medical Center	When compared to other scales, LAPSS had better specificity 88.7%, but had lower sensitivity (73.9%)
Rapid Arterial Occlusion Evaluation (RACE)	Face, arm, leg, language, gaze, neglect	RACE was published in 2013, and designed based on the NIHSS items with a higher predictive value for large vessel occlusion (LVO)	The scale has been validated in the field: RACE ≥5 scored by EMS predicts LVO with a sensitivity of 85% and specificity of 69%

(continued on next page)

Table 1
(continued)

Stroke Scales	Items Tested	Background	Characteristics
Others: The 3-Item Stroke Scale (3I-SS), Austrian Prehospital Stroke Scale (APSS), Shortened NIHSS For EMS (sNIHSS-EMS), Recognition Of Stroke In The Emergency Room (ROSIER), Acute Stroke Registry And Analysis Of Lausanne (ASTRAL), Los Angeles Motor Scale (LAMS), Prehospital Acute Stroke Severity (PASS), Vision, Aphasia, Neglect Assessment (VAN), Large Vessel Occlusion Scale (LVOS), Maria Prehospital Stroke Scale (MPSS), Melbourne Ambulance Stroke Screen (MASS), Medic Pre-Hospital Assessment For Code Stroke (Medic PACS)			
Scales Used in Hospital Settings			
National Institutes of Health Stroke Scale	Level of consciousness, extraocular movements, visual fields, facial muscle function, extremity strength, sensory function, coordination, language, speech, and hemi-inattention (neglect)	Developed in 1989 to assess differences in interventions in clinical trials. The modified NIHSS now consists of 13 items, following adjustments made from its original 15-item version	The NIHSS has established reliability and validity for use in prospective clinical research, and predictive validity for long-term stroke outcome

Glasgow Coma Scale (GCS)	Eye opening, verbal response, and motor response	First published in 1974 at the University of Glasgow by Graham Teasdale and Bryan Jennett	Useful as an outcome predictor in hemorrhagic stroke
Others: Canadian Neurologic Scale, European Stroke Scale, Scandinavian Stroke Scale			
Outcome Measure Stroke Scales			
Modified Rankin scale (mRS)	7 grades: 0 indicates no symptoms, 1 indicates no significant disability despite the symptoms, 2 indicates slight disability, 3 indicates moderate disability,4 indicates moderately severe disability, 5 indicates severe disability, and 6 indicates death	Developed in 1957 for assessment of stroke outcomes, and then modified in 1988 to improve its comprehensiveness	The mRS is considered responsive to changes in functional status after stroke. It is easy to implement and remains as the primary endpoint for many clinical trials
Barthel Index (BI)	The BI includes 10 activities of daily living (self-care and mobility). The normal score is 100, and lower scores indicate greater dependency	Introduced in 1965, by Mahoney and Barthel, as a measure of disability in people whose impairment interfered with independent use of their limbs	A number of studies have indicated excellent intrarater and interrater reliability for the BI
Others: Berg Balance Scale, Fugl–Meyer Assessment, Mini Mental State Examination, Montreal Cognitive Assessment, Beck Depression Inventory, Hamilton Depression Scale, Hachinski vascular dementia scale and Quality-Of-Life Scale (QOLS), Stroke Impact scale (SIS), Glasgow Outcome Scale, Functional Independence Measure			

Abbreviations: BE-FAST, balance, eyes, face, arm, speech, time; EMS, emergency medical services; FAST-ED, field assessment stroke triage for emergency destination; PPV, positive predictive value.

(CPSS). The best-performing scales were RACE, G-FAST, and CG-FAST with the highest area under the curve. It was considered that RACE, G-FAST, and CG-FAST outperformed other prehospital stroke scales because they incorporate both specific cortical symptoms (like gaze palsy and neglect) that are indicative of anterior LVO, and elements of the FAST test, which are highly effective in detecting LVO.[2] While other scales, such as PASS and C-STAT, also incorporate gaze palsy, they feature a more limited range of scores with fewer items. The authors concluded that even a minor 1-point change in scales with fewer items, such as PASS and C-STAT, could significantly affect their sensitivity and specificity when compared to scales with a broader range. A meta-analysis including 19 scoring systems from 13 studies aimed to determine the diagnostic accuracy of prehospital stroke scales detecting LVO. The results indicated that 3 scores, specifically the stroke Vision, Aphasia, Neglect (VAN) assessment, the NIHSS, and the LAMS, performed better in predicting LVO. This suggests that certain prehospital scoring systems, particularly those incorporating cortical signs, demonstrate better accuracy in predicting LVO.[12] In a retrospective analysis using data from the Safe Implementation of Thrombolysis in Stroke International Stroke Thrombolysis Registry (SITS-ISTR), researchers studied 3,505 patients focusing on those with complete NIHSS scores and documented vessel status. They found that the NIHSS item "best gaze" was strongly associated with LVO. All 3 components of the FAST test had high sensitivity in identifying LVO. Combining "best gaze" with the original FAST score (G-FAST) or high scores on other simplified stroke scales increased specificity.[13] While numerous validation studies have been published,[14–16] certain limitations persist, such as small sample sizes, exclusion of patients with posterior circulation stroke, intracerebral hemorrhage, or those without medical imaging. Moreover, substantial design variations make direct comparisons among these studies quite challenging. As stroke treatment indications expand, the use and implementation of prehospital scales to ensure the appropriate triage of these patients will become increasingly vital. Given the significant variation in organization and capacity among regional stroke systems of care, EMS personnel and local stroke champions should collaborate to identify the prehospital scales that best align with their specific regional stroke triage pathways.

National Institutes of Health stroke scale

The NIHSS (**Fig. 1**) is the most widely used scale globally, and the authors will discuss it separately in this section. It is noteworthy that this scale is also referenced in discussions of prehospital scales and included as part of stroke outcome measures. This reflects its application in a variety of clinical contexts.

The NIHSS was originally developed to assess variations in interventions for clinical trials, but its application has significantly broadened in patient care. It is commonly used as an initial assessment tool, for continuous monitoring of hospitalized stroke patients, and for planning post-acute care disposition. The scale has demonstrated both reliability and validity for prospective clinical research and predictive validity for long-term stroke outcomes.[17,18] It correlates well with both ischemic and hemorrhagic stroke volumes.[19,20] The scale is also reliable among providers with varying levels of medical training, even after relatively brief training in all aspects of the scale.[21] The NIHSS has been validated as an appropriate tool to evaluate and triage acute stroke patients remotely.[22,23]

Pitfalls

The NIHSS has been criticized for its complexity.[24] It is weighted to assess anterior circulation (AC) symptoms, which may lead to a reduced identification of posterior circulation (PC) strokes and potential withholding of treatment in such cases.[25] Of the

NATIONAL INSTITUTES OF HEALTH STROKE SCALE (NIHSS)	
1a: Level of Consciousness (LOC)	0 = Alert; keenly responsive 1 = Not alert; but arousable by minor stimulation 2 = Not alert; requires repeated stimulation 3 = Unresponsive, or responsive only with reflex
1b: LOC Questions	0 = Both answers correctly 1 = Answers one question correctly 2 = Answers neither question correctly
1c: LOC Commands	0 = Performs both tasks correctly 1 = Performs one task correctly 2 = Performs neither task correctly
2: Best Gaze	0 = Normal 1 = Partial gaze palsy 2 = Forced deviation
3: Vision	0 = No visual loss 1 = Partial hemianopia 2 = Complete hemianopia 3 = Bilateral hemianopia (including cortical blindness)
4: Facial Palsy	0 = Normal symmetrical movements 1 = Minor paralysis 2 = Partial paralysis 3 = Complete paralysis of one or both sides

5: Motor Arm
    5a. Left arm
    5b. Right arm
	0 = No drift
	1 = Drift
	2 = Some effort against gravity
	3 = No effort against gravity
	4 = No movement

6: Motor Leg
    6a. Left leg
    6b. Right leg
	0 = No drift
	1 = Drift
	2 = Some effort against gravity
	3 = No effort against gravity
	4 = No movement

7: Limb Ataxia	0 = Absent 1 = Present in one limb 2 = Present in two limbs
8: Sensory	0 = Normal; no sensory loss 1 = Mild-to-moderate sensory loss 2 = Severe to total sensory loss
9: Best Language	0 = No aphasia; normal 1 = Mild-to-moderate aphasia 2 = Severe aphasia 3 = Mute, global aphasia
10: Dysarthria	0 = Normal 1 = Mild-to-moderate dysarthria 2 = Severe dysarthria
11: Extinction and Inattention	0 = No abnormality 1 = Visual, tactile, auditory, spatial, or personal inattention 2 = Profound hemi-inattention or extinction
Total score= 0-42	

Fig. 1. Modified National Institutes of Health Stroke Scale. The figure includes 11 items and their scoring guide. (*Adapted from* the National Institutes of Neurological Disorders and Stroke.)

elements present on the current scale, motor function and cortical signs receive the highest punctuation. Symptoms such as limb ataxia and cranial nerve palsies receive fewer points and other PC findings such as truncal ataxia and nystagmus are not measured. Some evidence suggests that the NIHSS's validity in predicting outcomes is lower in patients with PC strokes compared to AC stroke patients.[26] When examining identical NIHSS scores, right hemisphere strokes have a larger median volume than left hemisphere strokes: Woo, and colleagues, reported that within each 5-point category of the NIHSS score below 20, the median volume of right hemisphere strokes was approximately twice that of left hemisphere strokes.[27] While the NIHSS is a strong predictor of stroke disposition and outcomes, it does not provide a complete assessment of an individual's post-stroke functionality. Therefore, the NIHSS is not well-suited for assessing various aspects of functional independence. The NIHSS should be used primarily as a quick assessment tool for stroke deficits and should not serve as a substitute for a comprehensive neurologic examination.

Stroke outcome measures

The care of post-stroke patients requires objective measurements of outcomes, which are crucial for assessing and evaluating treatment regimens. Various outcome measures have been suggested for evaluating strokes, spanning from widely accepted scales like the Glasgow Coma Scale, to more sophisticated systems such as the Disability Rating Scale. The utilization of these scales has been inconsistent, and clinical providers are uncertain about their relevance. The most commonly used scales to assess post-stroke outcome and disability include the Rankin Scale (RS), Modified Rankin Scale (mRS), Glasgow Coma Scale (GCS), Glasgow Outcome Scale (GOS), Barthel Index (BI), and National Institute of Health Stroke Scale (NIHSS). The GCS and NIHSS are commonly used to assist emergency personnel in selecting interventions, and to monitor acutely ill patients. These 2 scales lack the comprehensive evaluation tools required to measure an individual's functional performance. However, the NIHSS can be used to aid determining the degree of stroke severity. The BI continues to be widely used in clinical trials to measure outcomes, and the scale performs well even when interviews are performed over the phone.[28] In a study documenting the recovery of stroke patients, tracking their functional status before the onset of stroke, during rehabilitation admission, and at discharge, as well as outcomes 6 months post-discharge, Granger and colleagues found that patients achieving higher BI scores at discharge were more likely to reside in the community during follow-up. Among those living in the community, especially those with elevated BI scores, there was a reported increase in life satisfaction, more person-to-person contacts, and greater active involvement in community affairs.[29] The BI can be used to evaluate patients' improvement over time, and serves as a tool to determine the effectiveness of rehabilitative therapies.[30] The scale assesses various essential activities of daily living and specific physiologic deficits. However, it does not encompass many facets of functional independence, such as cognition, language, visual function, emotional impairment, and pain. Its "ceiling effect" has been noted, indicating that the highest score can be achieved by numerous disabled patients. This diminishes its effectiveness in distinguishing disability among individuals with higher levels of functioning.[31] Most patients will receive very low scores in the days immediately after the stroke. Therefore, the BI should not be used in acute stroke evaluations, as the scale is better suited to assess how individuals cope with their stroke symptoms.

The mRS is another extensively used stroke outcome scale. Known for its simplicity, it exhibits good stroke outcome validity and satisfactory inter-user reliability, particularly when a structured interview is implemented.[32] With a grading system ranging from 0 to 6 and broad categories within each grade, even a 1-point shift represents a clinically significant difference. In a prospective study involving 1530 patients 100 days after ischemic stroke, the mRS was found to be a superior instrument for distinguishing changes in mild-to-moderate disability compared to the BI, especially after mild strokes.[33] It is worth noting, however, that the scale's reliability diminishes when applied over the phone.[34] While the scale is used to monitor symptomatic improvement post-stroke, it should not be utilized at short intervals during acute hospitalizations, as patients may not have attempted to resume their regular activities. A recognized limitation of the scale is its lack of specificity. While it effectively captures how symptoms affect and are perceived by the patient, it does not objectively measure direct sources of disability. This limitation restricts the scale's ability to quantify the impact of interventions targeted at specific symptoms. Regardless, the mRS is frequently chosen as the primary endpoint to discern differences between interventions and plays a crucial role in the design of stroke clinical trials. Young and colleagues observed that mRS endpoints typically necessitated significantly smaller sample sizes to achieve adequate statistical power compared to BI endpoints.[35] Ordinal and dichotomized representations of the mRS have been compared, as slight differences in mRS grades could signify clinically significant changes. A dichotomy will miss meaningful improvements and might reduce statistical sensitivity for detecting differences between interventions.[36] Some authors have advised using ordinal approaches in trials analyzing the mRS, as this will detect more accurately long-term outcomes in stroke survivors.[37]

The Glasgow Outcome Scale (GOS) is another ordered scale. It has not been widely adopted due to its lack of detail, which limits its utility in both clinical practice and research.[38] While the scale is straightforward to implement, the GOS also exhibits greater reliability when conducted through a structured interview,[36] similar to the mRS.

Overall, there is a lack of agreement on the set of outcome measures to employ for evaluating physical recovery after a stroke. Choosing the suitable scales to assess stroke recovery proves challenging due to the diversity in stroke causes, symptoms, severity, and the nature of recovery itself. Certain limitations include the subjective nature of scale assessments, dependence on patient and proxy reporting, variability in application by health care providers, and limited sensitivity to mild clinical changes. Nevertheless, their overall value remains significant in both clinical and research settings.

Pitfalls

Stroke outcome measures are often comprehensive, time-consuming, and sometimes require direct observation, with the collaboration of the patient and/or their proxy. They do not correlate well with the stroke volume, and their inter-rater reliability can be affected when structured questionnaires are not implemented.[39] Nevertheless, reliable assessments that incorporate key aspects of functional independence and consider the perspectives of patients and/or proxies are essential to ensure effective rehabilitation for post-stroke patients.

SUMMARY

A comprehensive understanding of the availability and utilization of stroke rating scales is crucial for assessing stroke patients across the hyperacute, acute, and rehabilitation phases. These tools play a key role in treatment planning, outcome prediction, clinical monitoring, resource allocation, lifestyle adjustments, and rehabilitation strategies for stroke patients. Additionally, the scales are indispensable in the planning, execution, and comprehension of stroke clinical trials, having undergone thorough validation in both clinical practice and research. An effective stroke scale should exhibit both inter-obserever and intra-observer reliability. It should strike a balance between being comprehensive—encompassing relevant neurologic domains—and practical for ease of learning and rapid implementation in clinical settings. The scale should have high sensitivity and specificity for detecting neurologic symptoms. Additionally, it should demonstrate proven validity and applicability across international contexts. Every scale is unique and there is no one-size-fits-all solution. Scales that quantify neurologic deficits or specific bodily functions are commonly applied in the acute triage of stroke patients (including remote evaluations), and serve well for inpatient clinical monitoring. On the other hand, scales that assess post-stroke functionality, including patient's activities and reintegration into society, are often used to guide rehabilitation strategies.

FUTURE DIRECTIONS

On November 5, 1993, the National Institute of Neurological Disorders and Stroke organized a workshop to discuss the statistical approaches to the analysis of acute stroke trials with multiple prespecified outcomes, concluding that a global test was appropriate for ischemic stroke when no single outcome is accepted.[40] Given that a single scale does not measure all aspects of disability after stroke, an approach to integrate the scales using a global outcome statistical model had been proposed. A global statistical test is a method used in data analysis to assess the overall effect or impact of a treatment or intervention across multiple outcome measures or variables. Instead of analyzing each outcome measure individually, the global statistical test allows for the collective evaluation of the treatment effect across various rating scales. This approach enhances statistical power and provides a better understanding of the overall treatment efficacy.[41] This strategy should be considered potentially useful to determine the overall treatment efficacy for a combination of various stroke scales and could be regarded as a promising avenue for future research and clinical trials.

CLINICS CARE POINTS

- Documenting a prehospital stroke scale is recognized for enhancing sensitivity and positive predictive value in EMS stroke recognition.
- Outcome benefits of transferring stroke patients to a comprehensive center can are also be seen in ICH patients.
- Paramedics are encouraged to use some elements of the face-arm-speech-time test as an initial step for stroke symptom screening, as they prove highly effective in detecting LVO.
- The NIHSS is the most commonly used stroke scale. It was originally developed to assess variations in interventions for clinical trials, but its application has significantly broadened in patient care because of its excellent reliability, correlation with stroke volume, and validity to predict outcome.
- The BI continues to be widely used in clinical trials to measure outcomes, and the scale performs well even when interviews are performed over the phone.
- The mRS is widely used as a stroke outcome scale. It is simple, with high validity and satisfactory inter-user reliability. This is when a structured interview is implemented.

DISCLOSURE

The authors have nothing to disclose.

REFERENCES

1. Goyal M, Menon BK, van Zwam WH, et al, HERMES collaborators. Endovascular thrombectomy after large-vessel ischaemic stroke: a meta-analysis of individual patient data from five randomised trials. Lancet 2016;387(10029):1723–31.
2. Duvekot MHC, Venema E, Rozeman AD, et al, PRESTO investigators. Comparison of eight prehospital stroke scales to detect intracranial large-vessel occlusion in suspected stroke (PRESTO): a prospective observational study. Lancet Neurol 2021;20(3):213–21.
3. Nehme A, Rivet S, Choisi TJ, et al. Prospective evaluation of a two-scale protocol for prehospital large vessel occlusion detection. Prehosp Emerg Care 2022; 26(3):348–54.
4. Froehler MT, Saver JL, Zaidat OO, et al. Interhospital transfer before thrombectomy is associated with delayed treatment and worse outcome in the STRATIS registry (systematic evaluation of patients treated with neurothrombectomy devices for acute ischemic stroke). Circulation 2017;136(24):2311–21.
5. Goyal M, Jadhav AP, Bonafe A, et al. Analysis of workflow and time to treatment and the effects on outcome in endovascular treatment of acute ischemic stroke: results from the swift prime randomized controlled trial. Radiology 2016;279(3): 888–97.
6. Venema E, Groot AE, Lingsma HF, et al. Effect of interhospital transfer on endovascular treatment for acute ischemic stroke. Stroke 2019;50:923–30.
7. Brandler ES, Sharma M, McCullough F, et al. Prehospital stroke identification: factors associated with diagnostic accuracy. J Stroke Cerebrovasc Dis 2015;24: 2161–6.
8. DiBiasio EL, Jayaraman MV, Oliver L, et al. Emergency medical systems education may improve knowledge of pre-hospital stroke triage protocols. J Neurointerv Surg 2020;12(4):370–3.
9. Oostema JA, Konen J, Chassee T, et al. Clinical predictors of accurate prehospital stroke recognition. Stroke 2015;46(6):1513–7.
10. Dickson RL, Crowe RP, Patrick C, et al. Performance of the RACE score for the prehospital identification of large vessel occlusion stroke in a suburban/rural EMS service. Prehosp Emerg Care 2019;23(5):612–8.
11. Carrera D, Gorchs M, Querol M, et al. Revalidation of the RACE scale after its regional implementation in Catalonia: a triage tool for large vessel occlusion. J Neurointerv Surg 2019;11(8):751–6.
12. Vidale S, Agostoni E. Prehospital stroke scales and large vessel occlusion: A systematic review. Acta Neurol Scand 2018;138(1):24–31.
13. Scheitz JF, Abdul-Rahim AH, MacIsaac RL, et al, SITS Scientific Committee. Clinical selection strategies to identify ischemic stroke patients with large anterior vessel occlusion: results from SITS-ISTR (safe implementation of thrombolysis in stroke international stroke thrombolysis registry). Stroke 2017;48(2):290–7.
14. Noorian AR, Sanossian N, Shkirkova K, et al. Los angeles motor scale to identify large vessel occlusion: prehospital validation and comparison with other screens. Stroke 2018;49(3):565–72.
15. McMullan JT, Katz B, Broderick J, et al. Prospective prehospital evaluation of the cincinnati stroke triage assessment tool. Prehosp Emerg Care 2017;21(4):481–8.

16. Nazliel B, Starkman S, Liebeskind DS, et al. A brief prehospital stroke severity scale identifies ischemic stroke patients harboring persisting large arterial occlusions. Stroke 2008;39(8):2264–7.

17. Brott TG, Adams HP Jr, Olinger CP, et al. Measurements of acute cerebral infarction: a clinical examination scale. Stroke 1989;20:864–70.

18. Adams HP, Davis PH, Leira EC, et al. Baseline NIH stroke scale score strongly predicts outcome after stroke: a report of the trial of org 10172 in acute stroke treatment (TOAST). Neurology 1999;53:126–870.

19. Farooq S, Shkirkova K, Villablanca P, et al. National institutes of health stroke scale correlates well with initial intracerebral hemorrhage volume. J Stroke Cerebrovasc Dis 2022;31(4):106348.

20. Finocchi C, Balestrino M, Malfatto L, et al. National Institutes of Health Stroke Scale in patients with primary intracerebral hemorrhage. Neurol Sci 2018; 39(10):1751–5.

21. Goldstein LB, Samsa GP. Reliability of the National Institutes of Health stroke scale: extension to non-neurologists in the context of a clinical trial. Stroke 1997;28:307–10.

22. Berthier E, Decavel P, Vuillier F, et al. Reliability of NIHSS by telemedicine in non-neurologists. Int J Stroke 2013;8(4):E11.

23. Meyer BC, Lyden PD, Al-Khoury L, et al. Prospective reliability of the STRokE DOC wireless/site independent telemedicine system. Neurology 2005;64: 1058–60.

24. Dewey HM, Donnan GA, Freeman EJ, et al. Interrater reliability of the national institutes of health stroke scale: rating by neurologists and nurses in a community-based stroke incidence study. Cerebrovasc Dis 1999;9(6):323–7.

25. Libman RB, Kwiatkowski TG, Hansen MD, et al. Differences between anterior and posterior circulation stroke in toast. Cerebrovasc Dis 2001;11:311–6.

26. Inoa V, Aron AW, Staff I, et al. Lower NIH stroke scale scores are required to accurately predict a good prognosis in posterior circulation stroke. Cerebrovasc Dis 2014;37(4):251–5.

27. Woo D, Broderick JP, Kothari RU, et al. Does the National Institutes of Health Stroke Scale favor left hemisphere strokes? NINDS t-PA Stroke Study Group. Stroke 1999;30(11):2355–9.

28. Korner-Bitensky N, Wood-Dauphinee S. Barthel index information elicited over the telephone: is it reliable? Am J Phys Med Rehabil 1995;74:9–18.

29. Granger CV, Hamilton BB, Gresham GE. The stroke rehabilitation outcome study–Part I: General description. Arch Phys Med Rehabil 1988;69(7):506–9.

30. Mahoney FI, Barthel DW. Functional evaluation: the Barthel Index. Md State Med J 1965;14:61–5.

31. Kasner SE. Clinical interpretation and use of stroke scales. Lancet Neurol 2006; 5(7):603–12.

32. Wilson JTL, Hareendran A, Hendry A, et al. Reliability of the modified Rankin scale across multiple raters: benefits of a structured interview. Stroke 2005;36: 777–81.

33. Weimar C, Kurth T, Kraywinkel K. German stroke data bank collaborators. assessment of functioning and disability after ischemic stroke. Stroke 2002;33:2053–9.

34. Newcommon NJ, Green TL, Haley E, et al. Improving the assessment of outcomes in stroke: use of a structured interview to assign grades on the modified Rankin scale. Stroke 2003;34:377–8.

35. Young FB, Lees KR, Weir CJ. Glycine antagonist in neuroprotection (GAIN) international trial steering committee and investigators. strengthening acute stroke trials through optimal use of disability end points. Stroke 2003;34:2676–80.

36. Murray GD, Barer D, Choi S, et al. Design and analysis of phase III trials with ordered outcome scales: the concept of the sliding dichotomy. J Neurotrauma 2005;22:511–7.

37. Ganesh A, Luengo-Fernandez R, Wharton RM, et al. Oxford vascular study. ordinal vs dichotomous analyses of modified Rankin Scale, 5-year outcome, and cost of stroke. Neurology 2018;91(21):e1951–60.

38. Wilson JTL, Pettigrew LEL, Teasdale GM. Structured interviews for the Glasgow outcome scale and the extended Glasgow outcome scale: guidelines for their use. J Neurotrauma 1998;15:573–85.

39. Shinohara Y, Minematsu K, Amano T, et al. Modified Rankin scale with expanded guidance scheme and interview questionnaire: interrater agreement and reproducibility of assessment. Cerebrovasc Dis 2006;21:271–8.

40. Tilley BC, Marler J, Geller NL, et al. Use of a global test for multiple outcomes in stroke trials with application to the National Institute of Neurological Disorders and Stroke t-PA Stroke Trial. Stroke 1996;27(11):2136–42.

41. Pocock SJ, Geller NL, Tsiatis AA. The analysis of multiple endpoints in clinical trials. Biometrics 1987;43:487–98.

Moving?

Make sure your subscription moves with you!

To notify us of your new address, find your **Clinics Account Number** (located on your mailing label above your name), and contact customer service at:

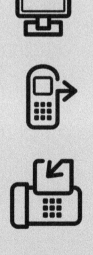

Email: journalscustomerservice-usa@elsevier.com

800-654-2452 (subscribers in the U.S. & Canada)
314-447-8871 (subscribers outside of the U.S. & Canada)

Fax number: 314-447-8029

Elsevier Health Sciences Division
Subscription Customer Service
3251 Riverport Lane
Maryland Heights, MO 63043

*To ensure uninterrupted delivery of your subscription, please notify us at least 4 weeks in advance of move.

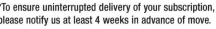

Printed and bound by CPI Group (UK) Ltd, Croydon, CR0 4YY

03/10/2024

01040473-0011